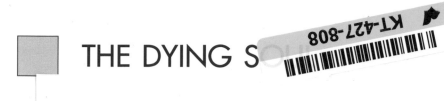

THE DYING S

FACING DEATH

Series editor: David Clark, Professor of Medical Sociology,
University of Sheffield

The subject of death in late modern culture has become a rich field of theoretical, clinical and policy interest. Widely regarded as a taboo until recent times, death now engages a growing interest among social scientists, practitioners and those responsible for the organization and delivery of human services. Indeed, how we die has become a powerful commentary on how we live and the specialized care of dying people holds an important place within modern health and social care.

This series captures such developments in a collection of volumes which has much to say about death, dying, end-of-life care and bereavement in contemporary society. Among the contributors are leading experts in death studies, from sociology, anthropology, social psychology, ethics, nursing, medicine and pastoral care. A particular feature of the series is its attention to the developing field of palliative care, viewed from the perspectives of practitioners, planners and policy analysts; here several authors adopt a multi-disciplinary approach, drawing on recent research, policy and organizational commentary, and reviews of evidence-based practice. Written in a clear, accessible style, the entire series will be essential reading for students of death, dying and bereavement and for anyone with an involvement in palliative care research, service delivery or policy making.

Current and forthcoming titles:

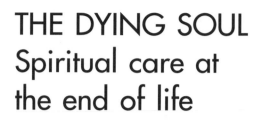

THE DYING SOUL
Spiritual care at
the end of life

MARK COBB

OPEN UNIVERSITY PRESS
Buckingham · Philadelphia

Open University Press
Celtic Court
22 Ballmoor
Buckingham
MK18 1XW

email: enquiries@openup.co.uk
world wide web: www.openup.co.uk

and
325 Chestnut Street
Philadelphia, PA 19106, USA

First Published 2001

A catalogue record of this book is available from the British Library

ISBN 0 335 20053 2 (pb)   0 335 20054 0 (hb)

Library of Congress Cataloging-in-Publication Data available

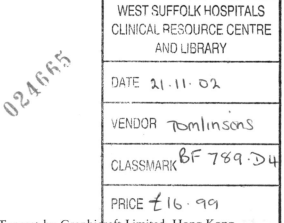
Typeset by Graphicraft Limited, Hong Kong
Printed in Great Britain by Biddles Limited, Guildford and Kings Lynn

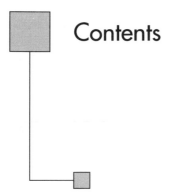

Contents

Series editor's preface

As the Facing Death series becomes well established, the scope of its interests is widening and deepening. We began with early volumes focused on the development of palliative care in Europe and around the world. These were concerned with matters of policy, with the recognition and need for palliative care service provision, as well as with some of the complexities of service delivery, audit and evaluation. A recent volume has been entirely devoted to the issue of research in palliative care. Another early focus has been on the personal and cultural experience of life threatening illness and of bereavement in which the authors have drawn on sociological and psychological perspectives to locate these issues within wider theoretical debates relating to the body, identity, gender and culture.

In the present volume Mark Cobb turns our attention to the question of spiritual care at the end of life. He is extremely well qualified for the task. Mark Cobb is an Anglican chaplain with several years' experience of working in hospitals and hospices. During this time he has developed a particular interest in palliative care and made important contributions to service developments, to teaching and to research in this field. He is widely known for his involvement in a series of conferences on the theme Body and Soul, which have explored the relationships between spirituality, religion and the delivery of health care. He is educated in the natural sciences and also in ethics, disciplines which enable him to bring a steady and analytic eye to his subject matter. At the same time his writing displays a warmth, a humanity and a compassion which is born of wide reading and generous reflection upon the nature of spiritual issues in the late modern context.

Why is this such an important book?

There are several answers to the question. *The Dying Soul* is a beautifully written, multi-faceted book which explores its subject matter from many perspectives. Running throughout is a willingness to tackle the vexed issue of what we mean by 'spirituality'. Here Mark Cobb is refreshingly prepared to forge a distinction between those aspects of human experience which constitute the *spiritual* and those which are better designated *existential*. In this he differs from some of his colleagues who prefer a less clear cut elision between the two and who thereby can run the risk of playing fast and loose with traditions within theology and philosophy that are quite distinct. In turn this raises the stakes on how 'the spiritual' can be cared for, particularly within the context of palliative care. For, as Mark Cobb demonstrates, spiritual care forms (at least rhetorically) part of a palliative care 'quadrilateral', the other components of which relate to the physical, the social and the psychological. So in opening up a space for the analysis of spirituality in this setting, he also makes us consider what we understand by the wider enterprise of palliative care, not least as it moves on from its roots in the hospice movement and the terminal stages of illness. Always he is eager to bring us back to social context, something which can get lost in the more inward and narrowly focused debates emerge in this evolving specialty. He is particularly strong in reminding us about death as an aspect of modern culture, the need to see palliative care as a force both responding to and also shaping that culture, and above all the permeability of those aspects of human experience which biomedicine prefers to separate into hermetically sealed zones. And all this in a wider context of discussion about the alleged 'secularization' of society and indeed of hospice and palliative care itself.

Many readers are now following the Facing Death series with enthusiasm and commitment. It is becoming an essential source for clinicians, social scientists, service planners and policy makers who appreciate that the care of those with life threatening illness and the understanding of human mortality are enterprises which are fundamentally intertwined. In doing this we are trying to move understanding beyond that which compartmentalizes these issues into matters of 'epidemiology', 'clinical care', 'policy' or 'theory'. It is an exciting and intellectually challenging approach. Mark Cobb's contribution here, in line with others in the series, is of vital importance in moving forward our understanding.

David Clark

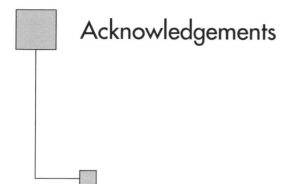

Acknowledgements

This book is written by one person but it is the result of my encounters with many. Clinical experience, teaching, conferences and many other forums have provided me with opportunities to learn from others, shape ideas, test arguments and express thoughts that would otherwise have remained a soliloquy. Among this crowd I must acknowledge and thank those who have had a direct hand in producing this book. First and foremost, Keith Arrowsmith warrants special acknowledgement and my gratitude for going beyond the call of duty by assisting me in so many ways throughout the writing of this book. David Clark deserves my particular gratitude for sharing in my early thoughts about this book and encouraging me in its writing. Likewise, Joanna Hocknell who cast her experienced eye over early drafts of chapters and provided me with an expert second opinion on particular matters. Although writing is a solitary task I am grateful to former colleagues at the Nightingale Macmillan Unit in Derby and present colleagues at the Trent Palliative Care Centre in Sheffield who have in many ways provoked and enriched my ideas about spiritual care and allowed me the space to develop them. Finally I am indebted to all those who have had to bear the cost of my writing and who have responded with patience, support and understanding.

Grateful acknowledgement is made to J.M. Dent for permission to reprint an excerpt from 'The Absence' from R.S. Thomas's *Collected Poems 1945–1990* and to Faber and Faber Limited for permission to reprint 'Siesta' from *The Eyes* by Don Paterson.

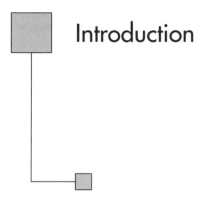

Introduction

The palliative care quadrilateral

The spiritual domain is routinely asserted as an integral part of palliative care alongside the physical, psychological and social aspects. This quadrilateral provides four views of an holistic philosophy of care and represents four interrelated ways of approaching the relief of suffering and the promotion of human well-being. This plausible convention is not without difficulties, particularly when we pay attention to the spiritual domain. To begin with, the term 'spiritual' is notoriously vague and obscure, yet widely used. It seems to provide a way of addressing something fundamental about humanity but remains abstract. In the past this openness was given a framework and orientation through Christianity. Today there is an insistent separation of the two. When we consider the practical matter of how the spiritual can be cared for, there is a range of responses that involve, to a lesser or greater extent, religion, psychology and aesthetic sensibility. Spirituality dissociated from a unitary belief system relies upon an eclectic mixture of ideas and philosophies. Further difficulty is added when questions of training, expertise and authority are raised: who should be providing spiritual care and what does this entail?

> Where there is sorrow there is holy ground. Some day people will
> realize what that means. They will know nothing of life till they do.
>
> (Wilde 1986: 143)

Spiritual care is written into the constitution of hospice and palliative care services and yet it remains the least explored and understood aspect. One reason for this is that when people contemplate the end of life they often find themselves having to look beyond the facts. The meaning and value of death transcend empirical reality and we can find in death a glimpse of the sacred which is both awesome and fascinating. If we find something of the sacred in death, then in approaching death through suffering and sorrow we may find ourselves having to walk on holy ground. Perhaps we do not or cannot take this step or we find the meaning of death sublime but inexpressible; either way there is an inevitable silence whenever we approach the sacred. However, this does not prevent us from exploring this domain and considering the very real questions of what all this means for the practical tasks of palliative care.

This, then, is the project of this book: to explore the familiarly unknown fourth side of the palliative care quadrilateral which is a way both of understanding and of responding to the spiritual dimension of being human. I have written out of my experiences as a hospice and hospital chaplain alongside an academic study of the subject. I therefore consider both theory and practice set within the wider contexts of health care and society. What will become quickly evident to the reader is that this is a field which readily spills out onto so many other fields. The reader will therefore find references well beyond the obvious subject matter and I readily draw upon a wide range of sources from the humanities and science. This book is written, therefore, to engage with readers in a number of different ways about the spiritual aspects of living, dying and death. Crudely, I take two approaches. Firstly, I write from the position of someone who takes the spiritual dimension of life, both embodied and intangible, as part of reality, and that '[a]lthough we seem to have an innate tendency to experience the natural in terms of the supra-natural, we are nevertheless under no compulsion to do so' (Hick 1999: 37). In doing so I take account of this aspect of human life at face value. Secondly, I write from the more distant perspective of the explanations and descriptions of spirituality proposed by various academic disciplines. The naturalistic theories provide empirical discourses and accounts of the spiritual phenomena in terms of human constructs, both individual and societal. Other perspectives study what is before them, tracing the surfaces and shapes of spirituality in order to provide clear descriptions. This analytical approach seeks to advance a better grasp of its subject without necessarily venturing to uncover hidden meanings or disprove the claims of a spiritual dimension. It will be evident that I work with both these approaches and take questions from one to the other in what I hope is a useful and creative attempt to bridge what is often considered something of a divide.

Questions of spirituality inevitably return us to questions about the nature and meaning of life. These are questions that are at the very heart of our existence and it is no surprise to find scientists alongside philosophers involved in attempting to explain such mysteries. In particular, the questions relating to consciousness, self and other mind/body problems (Damasio 1999) cause us to consider a fundamental question as to whether reality can be entirely accounted for by materialism. If it can be, then we may logically conclude that:

> the notion of an immaterial entity, of something thus outside of this domain, of something not directly observable, is viewed as a kind of intellectual violation and as a holdover from a less sophisticated era of human understanding.
>
> (Nicholson 1997: 31)

If, however, we consider reality to be broader and richer than this view allows then the material account is limited and we must search for other ways of making sense of and finding meaning in life. The spiritual dimension is what I generally take to refer to those aspects of the transcendent nature of reality which are part of human experience and which point beyond the material world. It is when we contemplate the end of life and face death that many people are aware of this dimension. This is because questions of our existence relate so closely to what we understand by death. The world faiths offer widely accepted perspectives on these universal questions, and Christianity in particular has been central to western thought on these matters. Yet we must also acknowledge approaches to these questions which do not rely upon an appeal to the transcendent or to theology but are broadly based in what can be considered the humanist philosophy of existentialism:

> We are all men hanging on the thread of a few rapidly vanishing years over the bottomless pit of death, destruction, and nothingness. Those objective facts are starkly real. Let us not try to disguise them. Yet I find it marvellously interesting that man's *consciousness*, his reason and his passion, can elevate these routine, objective, external events, in a moment of lucidity and feeling, to the status of a personally appropriated ideal – an ideal which does not annul those objective facts, but which *reinterprets* them and clothes them with the apparel of *man's subjectivity*.
>
> (Klemke 2000: 197)

The spiritual perspective, I contend, is distinct from the existential perspective in that although the latter allows for subjective transcendence it does not look beyond the 'universe of human subjectivity' (Sartre [1946] 1997: 55). This differentiation is readily overlooked in palliative care when the two perspectives are collapsed into a generic category that is a coverall for anything other than the physical, psychological or social. Another area of confusion and contention can be found in the use of the emotive phrase 'the sanctity of life' which is employed with reference to euthanasia and which resonates with a notion of the spiritual. The conviction that life is valuable and that it should not end prematurely seems to be a generally held view.

But the intrinsic value of human life can be understood in different ways, for example by appealing to the wonder of creation in either the evolutionary or the theological sense. It is wrong to assume that 'the sanctity of life' always refers to a religious doctrine and it cannot be presumed that it necessarily implies a spiritual perspective.

It will now be apparent that in approaching a book about spiritual care there is much weight that has to be borne repeatedly by a single word. Language enables us to communicate information and meaning. Sometimes the words we use are inadequate for what we try to convey, sometimes they are inaccurate and misinform, and sometimes we use words which no longer mean what they originally meant and there is uncertainty. Language is highly fluid, but it is also a vast repository of history: it is the place not only for creativity and novelty but also for convention and tradition. When we talk of the 'spiritual' we allude to a profusion of meanings, references and ideas. It is most obviously the currency of many religions. The humanities readily use the term and it has become a description of life's less tangible aspects. The spiritual is therefore a term from which can be inferred a vast range of meaning, some of which I allude to in this book and some of which the reader will bring to the text.

Spiritual care, pastoral care and Christianity

> What I think is upon us with the advent of the modern hospice is a counter-revolutionary movement – albeit modest – that nevertheless takes its stand against a secularized, impersonal, utilitarian and increasingly hostile world. What makes hospice philosophy or practice problematic for some is that many within hospice or the caring professions profess humanistic rather than traditional religious beliefs and in this post-Samaritan world find it difficult to acknowledge the fount of spiritual insight that guides and informs our actions. Many of us are thus conflicted and find it difficult to articulate a totally satisfactory philosophy for either our work or our lives.
>
> (Fulton 1986: 155)

The image of the hospice movement united in militant stance against the mundane forces of a secular world lends itself to apocryphal accounts of the hospice history. Fulton's use of 'Samaritan' is a direct reference to the eponymous biblical story which he takes as a classic example and inspiration for the hospice movement. However, what is apparent from the proceedings of the Yale colloquium of 1986 at which Fulton was speaking is that there was considerable dissension about the place of Christianity in the care of the terminally ill and whether there can be derived from it a universal notion of the spiritual (Wald 1986). Strong disagreement also emerged in a

British working party set up to examine the impact of hospice experience on the Church's ministry of healing (Working Party on the Impact of Hospice Experience on the Church's Ministry of Healing 1991). Differences in theology and practice surfaced as this interdisciplinary and interdenominational group met to consider the nature of hospice, healing and care. The issue of a universal or an exclusive spirituality appeared to be a particularly contentious matter and reflects a long-standing debate about what are the boundaries of the Church as a community. This difficulty is to some extent averted if, as the working party decided, the now familiar distinction is made:

> 'Spiritual' is often confused with 'religious'. Religious, however, means pertaining to a religion, i.e. a framework of theistic beliefs and rituals which give expression to spiritual concerns. While everyone has a spiritual dimension, in Britain today only a minority practise a formal religion. Hence, although people commonly say, 'I am not religious', they do not say 'I am not spiritual'.
>
> (Working Party on the Impact of Hospice
> Experience 1991: 151–2)

The problem of religion in palliative care is symptomatic of wider cultural issues. Religion is not abandoned, it is gradually relocated, and in its absence we are left with a spirituality not orientated towards God or the institution of the Church, but towards humanity and the organization of care. This can be traced from the social context in which hospice and palliative care has developed as well as from changes taking place within Christianity. In particular it is important that we recognize that spiritual care did not spontaneously materialize as the solution to a sudden problem but emerged to some extent from the direction followed by pastoral care (Wright 1996).

In the postwar period leading up to the opening of St Christopher's Hospice in London, the insights of psychotherapy and counselling were increasingly influential upon Christian theology and ministry. In the USA, the clinical pastoral education movement, founded by Anton Boisen, came to be a 'dominating force in pastoral care education within and outside the theological schools' (Gerkin 1997: 65) some of which crossed the Atlantic. In Britain similar developments were taking place, most notably in the establishment of the Westminster Pastoral Foundation and the Clinical Theology Association. Inevitably this was also a period in which pastoral care moved towards being more professionally organized and recognized as a specialist or 'expert' form of ministry: something evident in the institutional role of the chaplain. The scene was gradually set in the following decades for pastoral care to become transposed from a faith community to a health-care organization where humanistic elements could be readily appropriated as relevant to all people. The spiritual could thus exist without an explicit theology: a contrast that is illustrated in the following definitions.

> pastoral care . . . [is] the healing, sustaining, guiding, personal/societal formation and reconciling of persons and their relationships to family and community by representative Christian persons (ordained or lay), and by their faith communities, who ground their care in the theological perspective of the faith tradition and who personally remain faithful to that faith through spiritual authenticity.
>
> (Goodliff 1998: 10)

> spiritual care . . . [is] responding to the uniqueness of the individual: accepting their range of doubts, beliefs and values just as they are. It means responding to the spoken or unspoken statements from the very core of that person as valid expressions of where they are and who they are. It is to be a facilitator in their search for identity on the journey of life and in the particular situation in which they find themselves. It is to respond without being prescriptive, judgmental or dogmatic and without preconditions, acknowledging that each will be at a different stage on that personal spiritual journey.
>
> (Stoter 1995: 8)

If we can trace a line between these two modes of care it will be when the individual and the Christian community enter into dialogue, seeking connections between their stories and finding ways of interpreting each other's position. Because Christianity remains embedded in the cultural background of society and provides people some orientation for their beliefs, then this dialogical relationship may exist to varying degrees. For the person without such an orientation, pastoral care as defined above is rightly to be considered an imposition unless invited. Spiritual care overcomes this difficulty, despite its close relationship to pastoral care, because it faces away from a faith tradition towards the individual and does not seek to return. Therefore the individual's awareness and experience become normative within a permeable frame of reference constructed to some extent on-site.

Spiritual care is now a well established concept in palliative care, however ambiguous, where it clearly fits within the notions of individualized and holistic care. Spiritual care also provides a credible face to a society in which many faith traditions are represented and where many people are increasingly unfamiliar with any belief system. What is perhaps less certain are the ways in which spiritual care is actually implemented. There is currently a paucity of published descriptive research or accounts of practice, and so a normative approach cannot be presumed. I have therefore chosen to set much of my enquiry into the practice of spiritual care within an ethical framework which I take as applicable across all modes of care. This will allow us to consider particular claims of practice as well as the more fundamental issue of the place of spirituality in palliative care.

The book in outline

This book can be considered as falling into three sections. The first three chapters consider the concepts and theories that relate to spiritual care and the following three are concerned with matters of practice. The final chapter provides a summary of all the major themes dealt with in the book and draws from them directions for the development of spiritual care. What will become evident is that in looking at spiritual care we find ourselves having to attend to the overlapping frameworks of other discourses and the wider social context in which palliative care is embedded.

Chapter 1 is intended to provide an introduction to the vast subject of spirituality as it is understood and conceptualized from a variety of perspectives. I address specifically the nature of palliative care spirituality and suggest that there is a confusion between the generic use of the term and the heterogeneous nature of the spiritual. It may be considered that the spiritual dimension readily conforms to an holistic philosophy of care and yet it seems inconsistent with the approach of clinical science. I therefore consider the claims of medicine as they challenge spirituality and the meaning of dying and death. I suggest that a dissatisfaction with materialism and the widely reported experience of people support the notion of transcendence as a significant key to the nature of spirituality. This leads us into the contentious idea of the human soul which expresses for some the idea that we may transcend even death. Finally I set out the challenge which spirituality places before palliative care, both in the way it has become neglected and negated as well as in the way it is understood as part of well-being and suffering, life and death.

The spiritual is experienced and expressed in many ways, and I consider some of these in Chapter 2. Religious traditions of spirituality persist in an age where many do not actively participate in faith communities. I therefore explore the phenomenon of religion in contemporary society and its influence upon the way we face illness, suffering and death. To do this I take a multidimensional view and consider some of the major theories advanced to explain religion. I then sketch the religiously diverse terrain of Britain and the issues this raises for palliative care services. The secular argument is one that sees religion as outmoded and redundant, but there is sufficient evidence that religion is responsive to culture and therefore more prevalent and dynamic than predicted. This is no more apparent than in New Age religions which I consider as a paradigm of detraditionalized religion. However, the social and cultural transitions which have reshaped religion have also influenced how we care for the terminally ill. I end this chapter by drawing some analogies between palliative care and New Age religion, noting that contemporary expressions of the spiritual permeate palliative care both in terms of philosophy of care and in practice.

Dying has traditionally been viewed as a spiritual activity as much as a physical event. The modern hospice movement has attempted to reaffirm this aspect in the face of the grim postwar experiences of many in a predominantly curative healthcare system. In Chapter 3 I consider the spiritual significance of death and explore some of the major ways in which philosophy has tried to explain the nature of death. Death is symbolic of a range of meanings, some of which represent a complete ending and some of which point towards an ultimate destiny. I suggest that people's attitudes and approaches to death depend in part upon their beliefs, which include for many a spiritual dimension. Beliefs help to structure our worldview and can enable us to make sense of loss and find meaning in it. Yet few palliative care professionals consider these matter in their training or practice. One area that cannot be avoided is the rituals of death which are ubiquitous in health care. Rituals enact meaning, which around death can transform the cessation of life into a sacred event. They also point many people beyond death, and I consider some of the explorations that have been advocated of what happens after death. Finally I assert that the spiritual dimension of death is significant to bereavement and should not be disregarded by palliative care services in the support they offer.

In Chapter 4 I consider the contentious subject of who cares for the spirit. If palliative care claims to offer holistic care and to recognize the spiritual dimension then it is not unreasonable to expect that a service is capable in some way of responding to spiritual need. I therefore explore the notion of need in terms of spiritual care, particularly in terms of promoting the patient's good. In response to need, most palliative care services count a chaplain as part of their multidisciplinary team. I examine the role of the chaplain in providing spiritual care to patients and the wider roles that involve those people significant to patients, the staff and the service as a whole.

Spiritual care is also considered an aspect of the nurse's role, and I examine the claims and evidence for this both conceptually and in practice. I advocate that spiritual care is not a general obligation in a team and requires that responsibilities are specifically identified to avoid ambiguities and confusion. I also challenge the assumption that spiritual care happens inevitably in palliative care despite apparent uncertainty within some professions as to what this means. In conclusion I consider an interdisciplinary approach that provides an example of developing enhanced and integrated spiritual care.

Spiritual care is a defining and distinctive aspect of palliative care which, in Chapter 5, I consider from the organizational perspective. To begin with I examine the moral case that spiritual care should be intrinsic to palliative care in promoting the whole of the patient's good. If it is intrinsic then it must be practised with due regard to an ethical patient/carer relationship, but it also becomes an aspect of a managed organized service. The idealism of the vision in palliative care, the focus on performance and the measurement of outcomes are all considered. This leads me to suggest that a process of assimilation has taken place in palliative care that has had an impact upon the spiritual such that it may be reduced to a function of utility. Finally, I recognize that palliative care has become an increasingly mobile philosophy which is influencing practice in diverse settings and is itself being influenced by new demands. I therefore discuss some of the challenges that arise when spiritual care is considered in the contexts of acute hospitals and community care as well as with people of different faiths and people with non-cancer diagnoses.

Spiritual care cannot lie outside of the moral compass of health care and I therefore consider the issues of training, competence and accountability in Chapter 6. I begin by exploring whether or not spiritual care warrants professional practice and consider the claims of what it means to be professional. I suggest that if spiritual care is to contribute to more than a general sense of well-being then it should be established upon a professional ethic. This provides the grounds for practice which benefits patients and therefore fosters trust.

Inevitably, in exploring the issues of professional practice in spiritual care wider debates in health care are disclosed concerning the nature of orthodox practice, the grounds for therapeutic interventions and the moral nature of care. I argue that if spiritual care is an important aspect of palliative care then it should be done well and there should be some definition of what this means. A standard of spiritual care is provided as an example of promoting good practice. Despite a number of important caveats, I suggest that standards may help spiritual care to become more consistent, purposeful and integrated. Finally in this chapter I consider the inadequacy of training in spiritual care and propose that a range of knowledge and skills is necessary to respond to levels of competence appropriate to need. In addition to rigorous education I advocate that the provision of good spiritual care also requires adequate professional formation and the discipline of reflective practice.

Chapter 7 summarizes and reviews what I understand to be some of the key themes discussed in this book which affect the development of spiritual care. In each section I critically examine arguments and focus the challenges that they present. In the concluding section I note that spiritual care is replete with assumptions but short on creative dialogue and critique. Consequently I suggest three areas that need addressing in order to provide some direction to spiritual care. First, there is the neglected area of rigorous research which is crucial in developing some form of an evidence base. Spiritual care has been subject to very little study to ascertain either the nature of practice or the perspective and experience of patients. Second, there is the need to expand the knowledge base of the spiritual aspect of palliative care. This is not a unitary field of study but covers a range of academic disciplines. However, extant sources of knowledge and the knowledge of palliative care experience may provide a rich interdisciplinary source for critical enquiry given effective opportunities and support. Third, there is the need to develop the practice of spiritual care. Training health professionals is a key issue and I suggest that cognitive and behavioural modes of learning are complemented with experiential learning that draws upon an expanding research and knowledge base.

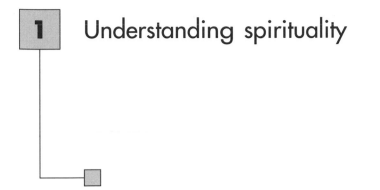

1 Understanding spirituality

Spirituality represents something of a conundrum. It is a term both ancient and modern, an anachronism and a contemporary issue. It occupies an increasingly popular space in western culture and yet is shrouded in mystery and ambiguity. Spirituality is to be found at the very foundation of the modern hospice movement, and it receives copious mention in palliative care, but it has no standard definition, practice or policy. There is a paucity of research about spirituality and few claim any expertise. And yet a concern for spirituality is one of the distinguishing features of palliative care, which prides itself in its holistic philosophy. Spirituality is apparently self-evident, but inscrutable, an unavoidable factor in dealing with suffering, dying and death but one which is elusive. It even has an inalienable place in the vocabulary of palliative care but is often referred to as a 'private' matter and therefore out of bounds for personal discussion.

There are a number of explanations that could be offered for this conundrum. A significant argument which we shall meet elsewhere in this book is that spirituality overlaps too much with religion, and religion is something that many people have become disaffected with. However, most people have not given up on their religious beliefs altogether; the problem then becomes one of how to find ways of describing and validating those beliefs outside of religious frames. Another well rehearsed explanation overlapping the first concerns the compelling claims of science. With a systematic world-view based on matters of fact, anything as undetermined as spirituality is easy to discount. Therefore, because palliative care trades to an increasing extent in the credibility of empirical science, spirituality must remain tacitly behind the scenes of this paradigm. pattern

A further explanation hinges upon the relationship we have with death and with the question of how should we die.

We live in a world that panics at this question and turns away. Other civilizations before ours looked squarely at death. They mapped the passage for both the community and the individual. They infused the fulfilment of destiny with a richness of meaning. Never perhaps have our relationships with death been as barren as they are in this modern spiritual desert, in which our rush to a mere existence carries us past all sense of mystery.

(Mitterrand 1997: vii)

Death frightens, fascinates, humbles and remains an outstanding enigma. How can we articulate the spiritual character of dying and death when the brutal facts of mortality cause such pain and anguish? How can we admit to the place of death in life when death contradicts so much of life and the expectations of death-defying health care.

Spirituality is an awkward subject to discuss, perhaps because we are all too close to it. The word can mean literally that which is of the essence of life, the animating breath, a vital and sustaining element of life. Talking personally about spirituality therefore requires people to become acquainted with and to lay bare their intimate thoughts and feelings. Spirituality consequently lends itself to metaphor, analogy, symbolism and art. It may be equally well described by saying what it is not. There are similarities here between spirituality and health. Health is hard to objectify, describe and measure; its absence less so, and it is readily concealed until disturbed. Spirituality, like health, is enigmatic and its familiar presence seldom registered until it is challenged or dislocated.

Despite its apparent abstruse and obscure character, spirituality as a term is frequently present in discussions about well-being, dying and death. In this sense, spirituality is closely linked to considerations of personhood. It is also applied to experiences of an esoteric or mystical nature, adding a significance of meaning and value. The playwright David Hare captures something of this in his play *Skylight*. Tom's wife has died from cancer, and in the following extract Tom expresses his grievance at his wife's spiritual feelings:

She got hold of this bloody word 'spiritual'. It's one of those words I've never quite understood. I mean, I've always hated the way people use it. They use it to try and bump themselves up. 'Oh I've had a spiritual experience', they say . . . As if that's the end of the argument. Spiritual meaning: 'it's mine and shove òff.' People use it to prove they're sensitive. They want it to dignify quite ordinary things. Religion. Now, that is something different. I like religion. Because religion has rules. It's based on something which actually occurred. There are things to believe in. And what's more, what makes it worth following – not that I do, mind you – there's some expectation of how you're meant to behave. But 'spiritual' . . . well, it's all wishy-washy. It means

'well for me, for *me* this is terribly important, but I'm fucked if I can
really say why . . .'

(Hare 1995: 44–45)

'Spiritual' for some is therefore a vacuous word because it is so bland or
unfathomable, made more elusive by being considered sacrosanct. It may
also suffer from being used in such a generic form that it has become too
malleable and therefore lost its distinguishing features. This points to a
further aspect of the conundrum: the ambiguity of spirituality and the
elusiveness of clarification. Spirituality therefore becomes a self-fulfilling
prophesy, respectfully ring-fenced and considered out of bounds to examination, research and exposition.

But is spirituality too fragile to withstand closer inspection or is it so self-
evident that it is innately understood? There are parallels here with another
popular palliative care notion, that of the 'good death'. This commanded
similar reverence and unquestioned assent as it achieved popularity in the
early history of the modern hospice movement. But through engaging with
it there has been a beneficial revision and development of what a 'good
death' means, and as a result palliative care has articulated more clearly not
only its aims but also its presumptions, values and ideals.

Being specific

It is evident that the term 'spiritual' requires some specification and the
benefit of points of reference. A simple map (Figure 1.1) of the conceptual
landscape that spirituality covers indicates something of the taxonomy
and lexicon which are circumscribed. These areas sometimes interrelate,
overlap and flow into one another. They can also be sharply divided and
contested. In palliative care the spiritual domain acquires a vague homogen-
eity simply because it concerns dying and death. The domain finds coherence
therefore around the motifs of human finitude, hope, suffering, wholeness
and destiny.

If, like David Hare's character Tom, the use of the word 'spiritual' incites
in you exasperation, attempts at definition, although not abundant, are
available. Many are found outside of palliative care in other contexts. One
such example comes from the American academic Nelson. In his study of
male sexuality and masculine spirituality he offers a broad account of spirituality which finds echoes in many others:

It is simply *our basic life orientations and the patterned ways in which
we express them*. It is the patterning of our thinking, feeling, experienc-
ing, and nurturing of whatever we take to be fundamentally important.

(Nelson 1992: 24)

Figure 1.1   Conceptual areas of spirituality

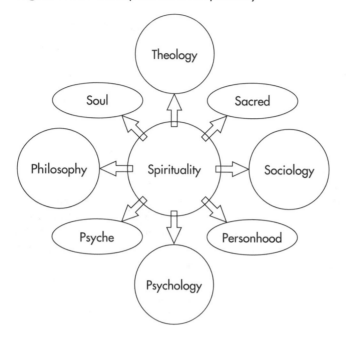

This definition captures some of the key 'components' of spirituality as it is commonly portrayed: spirituality is basic to being human and therefore something common to humanity; it gives shape and direction to life relative to essential principles, and is formative of, and in turn manifested in, being human. The qualification that it is what is held to be of *fundamental* importance is the critical determinant of spirituality. Nelson explains this to mean what is of ultimate reality and worth for a person; others use the phrase 'ultimate values'. However, whatever form these may take, content and their authorship are of equal significance. These may be developed or discovered, and range from an existential imperative of making meaning out of life to the 'reading' of universal values out of texts, traditions, the 'natural' order and supernatural revelations. And because these values are taken as fundamentally important they frame the 'world' which a person inhabits and are embodied by that individual in the way the person relates to life. In palliative care, spirituality acquires further definition by focusing upon the terminal orientation of life:

> The realisation that life is likely to end soon may well stimulate a desire to put first things first and to reach out to what is seen as true and valuable – and to give rise to feelings of being unable or unworthy to do so. There may be bitter anger at the unfairness of what is happening,

and at much of what has gone before, and above all a desolate feeling of meaninglessness.

(Saunders 1988: 1–2)

The unfinished business of the dying is a common idea which many views of spirituality complement (Dudley *et al.* 1995). At the hour of death, so convention has it, it is to be expected that people will want to have their lives in order, all outstanding matters resolved and their destiny clear. For patients who do not hold consoling beliefs about death, what faces them may be considered 'the obscene mystery, the ultimate affront' (Sontag 1991: 56) which is the cause of anguish, anxiety and emptiness. The spiritual task in palliative care is often portrayed, therefore, as that of finding meaning in death through which dying can be translated into the fulfilment of living, thus inspiring hope, wholeness and asserting the self in the midst of disintegration.

If death represents anomie and alienation of the individual, an authentic spirituality represents a means of personal growth and reintegration, in other words an aspect of psychological development (Bragan 1996). Psychology therefore offers a further detail to the complex spiritual map in recognizing the significance of belief (a sense of meaning) and faith (the capacity to believe) in the way that people face illness, dying and death (Jacobs 1998). Beliefs are ways of making sense of experience and exist on many levels and in many forms. Jacobs reminds us that 'Letting go at death is often just as much a psychological act as it is a physical one' (1993: 172), and that it is our beliefs which govern the way we understand and relate to death. This can have both negative or diminishing qualities, such as a crisis of faith, anxiety and doubt, as well as positive or enriching qualities, such as 'the courage to be' (Tillich 1952), trust and a sense of well-being.

A psychology of belief suggests that there is therapeutic potential in exploring matters of faith and belief with a patient. This potential is one that is recognized in some schools of counselling (Lyall 1995), pastoral care (Lake 1986) and psychotherapy (Jung 1933). No psychology of belief, however, can escape the imposing shadow of Freud, who wrote critically about why people hold beliefs. In one sense, Freud suggests that beliefs palliate reality, that they are consoling, may fulfil our (infantile) wishes and may be illusory. At his most critical, Freud held that religious beliefs serve to contradict and compensate for what he understood as the oblivion that follows death. But this conviction underestimates and misrepresents the richness of beliefs concerning death which address such issues as the significance of life, love, sacrifice, change, continuity, suffering and moral value (Bowker 1991).

Despite Freud's contempt of 'idolatrous' beliefs, people depend upon a wide range and level of beliefs in all aspects of life, even in psychotherapy, and the question of their truth endures ongoing debate and revision. In palliative care it is the beliefs not only of patients which are significant but also of caregivers, an area seldom explored. It seems remarkable that in a field that purports to be comfortable with death, that same field would appear to avoid exploring the beliefs which shape the way death is experienced, understood and cared for.

The ways in which psychological and physiological states are related deserve a brief mention because they provide a perspective on holistic care which can often be left to anecdote or discounted altogether. Psychological variables such as social support, beliefs and concurrent stress can not only influence the way in which patients cope with their illness but also affect their well-being. Psychological factors, as we have noted, also play their part in dying. There are many anecdotes of seriously ill patients surviving to celebrate wedding anniversaries, Christmas or birthdays and then dying. But there is also statistical evidence of significant fluctuations in mortality around the time of significant dates, such as religious festivals (Martin 1997). The findings of one study of three hundred patients cautiously conclude that the beliefs of a religious or spiritual nature are more predictive of clinical outcome in acute illness than the scores of the General Health Questionnaire (King *et al.* 1994). The proposed correlation between a course of illness and the nature and strength of a person's beliefs comes with many caveats, but it is a reminder that the process of dying is not just a matter of irreversible pathology and catastrophic biological failure for the individual or for society.

It would seem that no matter which angle we take on dying and death, there is in some inevitable sense a spiritual conjunction and even correlation. This in part is due to the silence of the rational enquiry as it stares at its demythologized death. But it may also be explained by the subjective experience and perception of mortality which takes us beyond death as an objective reality described within particular systems. The end of life may find an explanation in medicine, bereavement in psychology, dying in sociology, but death is not merely the resultant expression of these accounts. Death impacts upon us in the contemplation of our finitude, through our encounters with the dying and in the impress of their death. It therefore becomes a focus for beliefs, values, meaning and life itself. This is what has become in palliative care the category of spirituality, but it is a term that has acquired a putty-like malleability with its convenient gap-filling properties. It is not surprising, therefore, to find spirituality conforming easily to the holistic project such that it is claimed to be indispensable to quality care and 'the integrating aspect of human wholeness' (Clark *et al.* 1991).

This general comprehensiveness, which has become an indelible characteristic of palliative care spirituality, may sustain uncritical acceptance but it can obscure the significance of difference within spirituality both for professional caregivers and for patients. It is tempting, when faced with complexity, to try to circumvent it with some sort of unifying theory. But spirituality is represented and expressed in many different forms, no more so than in what might be called the 'religious spirituality' of the world faiths. Many of these forms contain concepts and assumptions which are incompatible with one another and cannot be brought together into a single account (Markham 1998). There are also differences within particular traditions apparent in the developments of divergent schools as well as more subtly in individual derivations. Spirituality is also in essence dynamic and easily distorted when reduced to a sketch of certain beliefs, values and practices that become a deterministic caricature – particularly evident in some multicultural approaches to palliative care (Gunaratnam 1997).

Palliative care spirituality can be understood as a collective term representing the assortment of spiritual orientations of patients, but it has also become a reflection of the 'common' spirituality that pervades the philosophy of much palliative care and which finds its origins in the modern hospice movement. In this latter sense, spirituality is grounded within a Euro-American context and is significantly influenced by Christianity and the western philosophical traditions. A 'common' spirituality should have no pretensions to being either a comprehensive global or a humanitarian account. Therefore spirituality used as a generic term is limited by its necessary abstraction, and limited in its direct application, but its contents may still have a broad significance and validity. A generic spirituality will be provisional, but it must hold some reliability otherwise it will be useless. Here there is a tension between pursuing the greatest degree of generality (simplicity) whilst maintaining what is particular and specific (complexity). But we must be aware also of a complacency that allows spirituality to be maintained as an ethereal mystery which can have the effect of obscuring enquiry, debate and specification.

Spirituality in palliative care must contain sufficient dependable detail and description to enable it to be recognized, understood and studied – the surface of the reality and its knowledge – whilst we remain aware that this will not capture the intimate and inchoate – the depth of the reality and its more profound discernment. Yet, through our underlying humanity and empathetic insight we can appreciate and, at times, comprehend this aspect of human experience in others. There is, however, an incompleteness to any account of spirituality, as in other attempts to portray and analyse human beings, such that:

> An immense amount is necessarily left out at both ends of the scale – both the deepest, the most pervasive categories which enter too much into all our experience to be easily detachable from its observation, and at the other end those endlessly shifting, altering views, feelings, reaction, instincts, beliefs which constitute the uniqueness of each individual and . . . the individual flavour, the peculiar pattern of life, of character, of an institution, a mood, and also of an artistic style, an entire culture, an age, a nation, a civilisation.
>
> (Berlins 1996: 19)

It is in this sense that spirituality is short of systematic theory and requires 'far more sympathy, interest and imagination, as well as experience of life, than the more abstract and disciplined activities of natural scientists' (Berlins 1996: 20). Although these quotations relate largely to historical theorizing, the argument retains validity for spirituality in that it also deals with the 'wholes' of people and their experience which are easily lost in analysis and derivation. It cannot be claimed that the description of someone by a biographer is equivalent to that of social scientist, or that their portrait is equivalent to their X-ray. Each has its use and value, but in each case the former representations are those of insight and acquaintance of the person whereas the latter are observations and the accumulation of particular data.

This presents a further paradox concerning spirituality, and again it is not one that is peculiar to it, for beyond its surface spirituality becomes increasingly unsusceptible to empirical and deductive techniques, although this still leaves a vast territory to explore and describe. The less we depend on assumptions and abstraction, the more we rely upon perception and awareness. It is perhaps not surprising, then, that some of the best language to convey the sense of spirituality is that of poetry, for it is at times necessarily analogical and metaphorical, often conforms only to sufficient grammatical rules to make it 'legible', and can by circumlocution and apophasis say much without direct reference to the subject. Poetry is perhaps *the* language of paradox, and so it is in the poetry of R.S. Thomas that we discover, for example, this simple but penetrating account of the need to pray:

> It is this great absence
> that is like a presence, that compels
> me to address it without hope
> of a reply. It is a room I enter
>
> from which someone has just
> gone, the vestibule for the arrival
> of one who has not yet come . . .

('The Absence', Thomas 1995: 361)

Thomas's ability to deal with the paradoxes of absence and presence, faith and doubt, provides the means to convey his search for what he believes to be ultimately real. Poetry may give our deepest thoughts, beliefs and experiences words, but it is not a medium which is commonly used in the commerce of logical discourse, and it is certainly not the common parlance of palliative care despite the inclusion of creative arts within the therapeutic context. The language of palliative care spirituality is therefore more often reliant upon second-hand languages that provide an impersonal perspective on a world that is intelligible but often lacks a sense of meaning, reason or value, those things which are often the loci of spirituality in what may be termed a 'disenchanted' world. Plainly we need a reliable account of spirituality, robust enough to be pragmatic and enable useful reflection and enquiry. This is not a mere semantic exercise, but one which requires spirituality to stand in a confident relationship to others who are sifting reality, contemplating being human and who are motivated to care for the dying.

Science, medicine and spirituality

The thought of putting science and spirituality together may at first appear a rather odd conjunction, for science deals in objective realism, and spirituality in the very soul of being. It could be said, therefore, that science looks in from the outside while spirituality looks out from the inside. But both approaches are trying to make sense of life and to respond to the human preoccupation with the nature of reality.

In his exploration of some of the latest scientific theories, George Johnson looks across from the cutting-edge science institutions of New Mexico to the local communities and traditions:

> The descendants of the Anasazi dancing in resonance with the seasons, the fundamentalists with their attempts to predict the future through biblical interpretation, and the physicists and biologists with their search for hidden harmonies are battling over the same spiritual ground. All are trying to make sense of life's overwhelming complexity, to come to terms with the fact that, for all our well-laid plans, we are buffeted about by contingency and chance. Each of these subcultures, in very different ways, is trying to replace randomness with order, to spin webs of ritual and reason, to try and convince itself that if we don't actually live at the centre of creation, at least we can comprehend it – that there is reason to believe that the human mind can pierce the universal panoply. Each is trying to answer the question of why we are here, as a species, a society, and as individuals. In both science and religion, we seek creation myths, stories that give our lives meaning.
>
> (Johnson 1995: 26)

This generous cosmological interpretation suggests a common purpose in the search for understanding and truth. At its most diplomatic, this inclusive view does not consider science and spirituality to be mutually exclusive. It allows accounts to co-exist because it does not allow for absolute claims to reality. As we shall see, when facing death there are few who would be so bold. However, some of the most powerful critics of this accommodating position come from within the scientific tradition, and particularly modern biology, where claims have been staked for the sole possession of the 'spiritual ground'. Richard Dawkins considers that natural selection outclasses all explanations of life and believes it to be a blind process with no purpose or meaning other than maximizing DNA survival.

In considering more personal matters, such as suffering, Dawkins is convinced that:

> In a universe of blind physical forces and genetic replication, some people are going to get hurt, other people are going to get lucky, and you won't find rhyme or reason in it, nor any justice. The universe we observe has precisely the properties we should expect if there is, at bottom, no design, no purpose, no evil and no good, nothing but blind, pitiless indifference.
>
> (Dawkins 1995: 133)

A universe of 'selfish genes' is a sufficiently complete explanation of life for some; other scientists question just how blind the evolutionary process is and point to its tautological weakness particularly in the circularity of evolutionary arguments. But for many it is hard to believe that an absurd chain of contingencies says all that needs to be said about humanity. The simple point is that science offers its explanations of the physical impersonal world it investigates and that this is not limitless, otherwise we have to concede that science has become omniscient, and that scientism is the order of the day. Scientific reductionism extrapolated to the corners of a multifaceted world also throws up a smokescreen to the questions it cannot answer, the values it has no use for, the purposeful beliefs it occludes with functional utility. We are left therefore with powerful tools and technology and yet as strangers in a cosmological drama in which we now appear in the margins, as one whose divine fiat is surplus to requirement. This is what is referred to as a disenchanted world (Weber), barren of the meaning, experience and understanding that science brands as fiction or fantasy. But that is seldom the personal and embodied world inhabited by human beings who, for example, experience pain and delight in ways that biology or physiology can hardly begin to describe.

Death reduced to an event of medical science was the starting point for the modern hospice counter-movement whose vision combined both the scientific and the spiritual. However, in the desire for credibility and status, palliative care is an uncomfortable position. For as it develops its own specialist clinical science, and returns increasingly to the place from which it departed – acute health care – it may have to abandon some of its distinct philosophy, and as a result the concern for the spiritual may become compromised or even relinquished (Small 1998). But this assumes that this goal is worth achieving and that the progress of science, and more specifically medicine, from which palliative care wishes to benefit, is at least benign and preferably rewarding. And yet as medicine has become more and more ambitious and dominant so too have its discontents and nonconformists.

Illich famously criticized the medical monopoly of health care for undermining people's ability to face the reality of illness and deal with sickness and death, claiming that the technocracy of medicine was eradicating the meaning of suffering. Pain for example, Illich argues, has become a term used almost exclusively to refer to bodily pain to be managed by external technique, whereas historically its meaning was cosmic, mythical and an experience as much of the soul as of the body. Therefore, pain was always more than reflex or dysfunction: 'there could be no source of pain distinct from pain that was suffered' (Illich 1976: 156). Disquiet with the medicalization of death has been paralleled with growing opposition to the prolongation of life, evident in the drive towards legitimizing euthanasia. Porter, from an historical perspective, recognizes that, for centuries, medicine could achieve little and therefore people had low expectations of it. In the twentieth century, medicine grew in its achievements, its status, cost and therefore its attractiveness to critics. In western society, medicine increasingly faces another plight, and one that will possibly dictate a more ignominious future:

> Having conquered many grave diseases and provided relief from suffering, its mandate has become muddled. What are its aims? Where is it to stop? Is its prime duty to keep people alive as long as possible, willy-nilly, whatever the circumstances? Is its charge to *make* people lead healthy lives? Or is it but a service industry, on tap to fulfil whatever fantasies its clients may frame for their bodies . . .
>
> (Porter 1997: 717)

The relationship between palliative care and medicine is a critical one, not only for the future of palliative care but also for the place of spirituality within it. If palliative care adopts an increasingly reductionist view of terminal illness and dying, it will come to operate with an increasingly impoverished understanding of those for whom it cares as well as those who provide the care. If it can continue to assert its distinctive philosophy and approach it may also continue to embrace a wholeness of human being, suffering and dying that is often obscured or even absent from the sparse view of science. The undoubted effectiveness of medical science must not distract us from its constraints, nor lead us to consign spirituality to a type of epiphenomenon which will eventually be dissolved by cognitive science.

Palliative care is embedded within a wider culture in which science has radically transformed the concept of the self through its relentless materialism and revolutionized our understanding of reality through its reconstruction of the universe. In simple terms this can be traced as a shift from dualism to monism; from a world in which there were physical and spiritual domains to one dominated, to the exclusion of all else, by the purely physical (Wertheim 1999). But for many people this is neither adequate nor sufficient. The spiritual has not ceased to exist because there is no place for it in the scientists' construction of the world. One perspective cannot provide a comprehensive view of the totality or provide an 'absolute' knowledge; however, the fallacy is to assume that anything unaccounted for in science is simply obsolete, for 'a methodological limitation does not warrant the conclusion of a corresponding ontological poverty' (Polkinghorne 1996: 112).

The scientific imagination is the very opposite of impoverished, and through it medicine has transformed our expectations of life. But medicine's success has been at a cost, and part of that cost has involved a myopic view of illness as pathology, with its damaging consequences for practice. Palliative care, without abandoning scientific developments, has sustained a broader approach and integrated different perspectives that give high regard to the personal and social experience of illness. Perhaps it is because science has relatively little to say in the presence of suffering and death that spirituality still has a place in palliative care. A scientific account, for example, of the cessation of biological life is at best banal and does not capture the profound attitude most people express towards death evident in their response of grief. Again we come across the difference between the causal scientific objective explanation and the human subjective world of meanings and beliefs. This is why medicine and the science upon which it is based can be so alienating, but it may also be why:

> Those who seek for meanings may be indifferent to causes, and those who communicate with God through prayer should be no more cut off from him by the knowledge that the world of objects does not contain him, than they are cut off from those they love by the knowledge that words, smiles and gesture are nothing but movements of the flesh.
>
> (Scruton 1996: 107)

Transcendence and the nature of spirituality

A sense of alienation from the world and from one another points us towards the notion of transcendence which is perhaps becoming a significant attribute of spirituality today. Transcendence at its most literal is about going beyond the self, the body, the physical and the mortal. It is a term that can convey a sense of being a part of a greater whole, of connecting with something outside of oneself, or of becoming open to a greater reality that may be in the depths of one's being, with another person, with the world or with God. Common experiences of transcendence involve the awareness of an 'other' beyond the immediate and of losing oneself in its contemplation. Falling in love with another person, taking in a dramatic landscape, viewing a beautiful work of art or listening to music can all be occasions for transcending our selves as well as the object of our consideration. All this can be considered, therefore, in terms of an aesthetic experience or encounter:

For I have learned
To look on nature, not as in the hour
Of thoughtless youth; but hearing oftimes
The still, sad music of humanity,
Nor harsh, nor grating, though of ample power
To chasten and subdue. And I have felt
A presence that disturbs me with the joy
Of elevated thoughts; a sense sublime
Of something far more deeply interfused,
Whose dwelling is the light of setting suns,
And the round ocean and the living air,
And the blue sky, and in the mind of man:
A motion and a spirit that impels
All thinking things, all object of all thought,
And rolls through all things.

('Lines composed a few miles above
Tintern Abbey', Wordsworth)

Wordsworth's consecration of nature shifts the focus from the self to the other which lies beyond and outside the self but is experienced within. The beauty of nature for Wordsworth has this sublime reality in which 'we see into the life of things', something both perceived and revealed:

Enough of Science and of Art;
Close up those barren leaves;
Come forth, and bring with you a heart;
That watches and receives.

('The Tables Turned', Wordsworth)

In going beyond a description of landscape, Wordsworth senses the sacred in nature, that which is of ultimate value. In contemplating humanity, he sees 'Thou, whose exterior semblance doth belie Thy soul's immensity' such that we are not born 'in entire forgetfulness/And not in utter nakedness/ But trailing clouds of glory . . .'. This aesthetic interest, expressed in this case in romantic terms, engages our little world in a wider world of arresting allusion, spiritual significance and morality. And all this through reflecting on the ordinary, material, everyday world. Perhaps here is where the aesthetic and the religious converge in attempting to convey deeper truth:

In the sentiment of beauty we feel purposiveness and intelligibility of everything that surrounds us, while in the sentiment of the sublime we seem to see beyond the world, to something overwhelming and inexpressible in which it is somehow grounded. Neither sentiment can be translated into a reasoned argument . . . All we know is that we can know nothing of the transcendental. But that is not what we *feel* – and it is on our feeling for beauty that the content, and even the truth, of religious doctrine is strangely and untranslatably intimated.

(Scruton 1998: 29)

Existential uncertainty, dissatisfaction with materialism, the search for meaning and value almost compel transcendence. Thus we attribute awe and wonder, the sacred and the holy, to experiences of transcendence because they give a breadth to the world we inhabit and we become affirmed, consoled, and connected beyond the loneliness of ourselves. This has much in common with an 'oceanic' experience (attributed by Freud to the mother/baby relationship) in which a person feels at one with the world in an unbounded union. However, there is a mystical tradition, evident in many religions, that is far from infantile and understands the abdication of the ego as the way to being at one with the universe. Transcendence, therefore, can be understood as the disclosure and realization of significance beyond the particular. For those who hold religious beliefs, transcendence may involve an encounter with the natural through which the supernatural is experienced: a sacramental reality that makes present the 'ultimate reality' of God. This endows the world with a telos, or ultimate purpose, according to the religious hermeneutic and faith. Bond declares, however, that '[t]heology has lost its object' such that God 'has become pluralized into a general spirituality and identified with virtually anything whatsoever' (Bond 1998: 286). A telos without reference to God, or the supernatural, operates in the noumenal world rather than the empirical world, and transcendence becomes similarly abstract and indeterminate, an aesthetic sublimity without orientation or value. Thus we approach a major question in our understanding of spirituality: can spirituality exist without theology or without religious faith? Can there be a secular spirituality? These are question which, as we shall see, have been debated in palliative care as much as anywhere else.

Spirituality contains a tension, therefore, in that it is expressed and experienced in distinct forms and traditions, whilst also being taken as a unifying, although pluralistic, concept within which all people can be included equally. This patterns to some extent the sociocultural epithets of modernity and postmodernity, the latter suggesting a deregulated spirituality whose authority resides in the individual, rather than in any 'ultimate' truth or orthodoxy, with its resultant relativism. It is perhaps of some surprise that the idea of spirituality has survived at all given the claims of secular theories, but the secularization process is losing its confidence and becoming weakened by its limits. Counter-trends have helped to support spirituality, evident in the concern about quality of life and well-being, human rights, ecology and moral values. It is perhaps ironic that contemporary spirituality to some extent finds endorsement within the cultural sphere, and in areas not readily associated with it:

Consumerism, with its emphasis on taste, and the accompanying aes-theticisation of social life, along with the new centrality of what might be called a 'sacred self'; these may signal not only a new apprecia-tion of the symbolic realm but also offer opportunities for considering these 'religiously': that is, as evidence of a quest for transcendent meaning.

(Lyon 1996: 20)

The quest for meaning, the questions of existence, are pressing human preoccupations that people are motivated to address in some form or other, both individually and collectively. The survival or continuation of spiritual-ity may need to be thankful to the demythologized and disenchanted views of our world which claim such attention. But this is not to suggest a dicho-tomy or contradiction that requires a simple choice of alternatives; rather it is to recognize the dynamics of spirituality and its cultural embeddedness. It also reminds us of the enduring and inherent question put before us each morning as we stare at ourselves in the mirror, a question that is perhaps no more urgent than when life is fading: what is the 'me' that I see and which lives in this body? To use the more eloquent language of the seven-teenth century, which retains relevance for today, 'what is this quintessence of dust?' (*Hamlet*, ii.ii.306). A succinct reply may be found in one of Donne's Holy Sonnets, 'I am a little world made cunningly/Of elements and an angelic sprite.' (V.) And with that we turn to another significant concept for our understanding of spirituality, that of soul.

Soul

The spiritual connotations of soul have not limited its application to mat-ters such as music, friendship and food. Soul denotes something essential, noble and sincere; it is a word of some gravity and much historical signifi-cance. Indeed, its etymology takes us back at least to the foundations of western philosophy and theology, and yet its usage persists into contempor-ary debates about the nature of the self and consciousness (Crabbe 1999). One of the best examples is to be found in the Platonic dialogues of *Phaedo* (Gallop 1993) which concern Socrates on the day before his execution (399 BCE). The dialogues explore the nature not only of death but also of life after death, and presents one strand of an ancient Greek understand-ing of soul (Greek *psyche*) that was to have a major influence on Christian theology, and which can be perceived in common notions of soul prevalent today. A few examples will be illustrative:

'. . . tell me what it is, by whose presence in a body, that body will be living.'
'Soul.'

'And is that always so?'
'Of course.'
'The soul, whatever it occupies, always comes to that thing bringing life?'
'It comes indeed.'

(Gallop 1993: 105 c,d)

'. . . And that being dead is this: the body's having come apart, separated from the soul, alone by itself, and the soul's being apart, alone by itself, separated from the body? Death can't be anything else but that, can it?'
'No, it's just that.'

(64c)

'. . . if these are our conclusions from all that's been said: soul is most similar to what is divine, immortal, intelligible, uniform, indissoluble, unvarying, and constant in relation to itself; whereas body in its turn, is most similar to what is human, mortal, multiform, non-intelligible, dissoluble, and never constant in relation to itself.'

(80b)

Phaedo does not present a systematic theory of soul, and I am not suggesting that one is read into it, but we can see here the notion of soul as the animating principle (Latin *anima*), in some form of dualistic relationship to the body, and immortal upon the death of the body. However, there are considerable differences with a modern understanding of soul, for the Platonic soul has a prenatal existence, it operates in the mode of reasoning and intellectual function, and has a place in the metaphysical theory of forms which has long been abandoned (Gallop 1993). Despite the historical canyon and the unfamiliar world-view separating us, the Platonic ideas of soul have a remarkable contemporary resonance. Perhaps, dealt with simply, this is not so unexpected, for little has changed in the face of death when a sense of the body being abandoned is felt as much as the cessation of life is observed.

This points us to the thorny philosophical problem of whether or not a person can be subdivided into a collection of ontological 'components'. Is a person a unity, or is there a 'ghost' in the machine? Is the psyche (understood as mind) a product of the brain or an enduring and distinct entity? Cartesian duality has contributed greatly to the success of somatic medicine, but it has also left the door open for ways of reaching the soul. Thus Sacks, reflecting on postencephalitic and Parkinsonian patients, suggests that a practical scientific medicine must be complemented with 'an utterly beautiful and elemental "existential" medicine' (Sacks 1982: 241–55) that can deal with the 'I' as opposed to the 'It' and includes living contact and art. Others have gone a step further, and so in psychoneuroimmunology an attempt is made to bypass the duality by challenging the psychosomatic fallacy that says either disease is a physical reality or it is all in the mind and therefore 'imagined' – in its pejorative sense.

Perhaps the greatest challenge lies in the explanation of the nature of consciousness, the experience of the self, the subject which science attempts to translate into an object by describing it in terms of an epiphenomenon of matter or a cognitive mechanism (LeDoux 1998). In this materialist reduction people are no more than biological creatures, whose self is an erroneous and deceptive illusion. The hypothesis of memes suggests that 'I' is a clever trick of evolutionary natural selection which may be more harmful than benign, and that explains 'why we all live our lives as a lie, and sometimes a desperately unhappy and confused lie' (Blackmore 1999: ch. 17).

But the autonomous self is self-evident to many people and an immensely powerful notion in the way we think about ourselves, others and mortality. This may be why the language of soul is still in common use even if the elaborate metaphysics of Plato have been forgotten or displaced, for it still represents a significant aspect of personhood. In this sense, soul has associations with the value and dignity of life, its moral agency and its potential. Soul also retains an ethical purchase when entering debates regarding the sanctity of life, euthanasia and abortion. Here the soul symbolizes the core of human life, of intrinsic value to be respected and honoured, whether 'created' by a divine or an evolutionary process (Dworkin 1993: ch. 3). Therefore soul is in some sense a reflection of the fundamental values around which life is patterned and which gives life worth and fulfilment. The dynamic in this patterning is evident in the questing after the authentic self, never fully realized but a goal that fascinates and inspires:

> The longest journey
> Is the journey inwards.
> Of him who has chosen his destiny,
> Who has started upon his quest
> For the source of his being
>
> (Hammarskjöld 1964: 65)

Self-awareness suggests, intuitively at least, an inward gaze that goes beyond the surface persona to an intimacy with the self. This spatial analogy of the journey towards one's being is evocative of a 'world within' and accords with an internalized soul. But soul, as the pattern and goal of the self, may be thought of not as containing but as embracing the person. It is this concept of soul that brings us close to a metaphysics in which immortality and destiny can be contemplated. Transcending our limits may be an hubristic aspiration that can work against our humanity – escape and denial – or it may turn us to attend with more concern to this life, sometimes evident in the spirituality of palliative care. However the soul also provides the possibility of a continuity despite death, a hint of the eternal and something beyond mortal limits. These immortal longings have been the subject of grand philosophical and theological projects (Kerr 1997), but more simply the idea of soul equips people to look into the oblivion of death, to honour the dead and to afford care to the dying.

The language and symbol of soul clothes a complex of problems and phenomena pointing away from nihilism and towards an expression of being human that is inspiring, profound and transcendent. Perhaps this is why the word has become so embedded in our vocabulary and thinking, receiving the attention not only of certain branches of theology and philosophy (Morea 1997; Swinburne 1997) but also of cognitive science and psychology (Brown *et al.* 1998). It is a concept that both challenges and fascinates, no more so than when contemplating the end of life, suffering and human destiny. In this sense alone, soul retains an heuristic potential, even if the mythology of soul can be difficult to correlate with other types of discourse and is susceptible to criticism. Soul has historically provided a focus for the human experience of being in the world and a characteristic of life itself. This nexus has intersected for many with spiritual dimensions that enable us to talk about the transcendent capacity we have beyond our fragile and ephemeral bodies. Questions of the existence and place of a human soul, which seem to occupy more the thoughts of scientists than theologians and philosophers, lead to an important question of whether or not we can live and die without soul. It is a critical debate not only about what it means to be human but also about the value and meaning of human life. The importance of soul may therefore reveal itself by its absence in the accounts of humanity that diminish not only the individual self but humanity as a whole:

> The denial of the soul leads to loss of the ideal of individual worth; to loss of a sense of the absolute claims of love and truth; to loss of a real sense of moral purpose and the importance of moral striving in the world. If we are really to seek for justice and human freedom and self-realization for all, it is vital to recognize the human soul for what it is – the transcendent subject that is never wholly bound by the material forms in which it is, nevertheless, truly incarnate.
>
> (Ward 1992: 116)

The ethical framework suggested by Ward pivots upon the idea of soul which strives to find fulfilment in responding to absolutes of love, truth and justice – an objective moral basis whose goal is of ultimate value, namely God. This represents a particular theistic spiritual orientation which is influential in palliative care and provides a sense not only of moral dignity but also of moral obligation. The soul has not been left alone by other traditions: claims have been made upon it by other philosophies, and increasingly by science. These varying accounts do not represent equivalent understandings: some attempt to make others redundant, others conflict at their most elementary level, but to speak of the soul is an attempt to speak of something significant about ourselves and others, about human purpose, destiny and even our place in the life of the universe (Tilby 1992). Debate and disagreement naturally accompany such accounts, for they concern pressing matters, but what is apparent is that the soul is far from receding in the discourse of humankind despite a fading historical importance or any contemporary dissent.

The challenge of spirituality

It is apparent that spirituality has an enormous range of interpretations that include the theistic, non-theistic, atheistic, ascetic, moral, psychological and scientific. They all concern making sense of human existence. This is not the preoccupation of all people: some are content to accept life as it is and go no further. Whether people facing death consider such matters to a greater extent than others is open to speculation, but what is certain is that mortality has occupied an important place in the concepts and expressions of spirituality. If spirituality concerns the significance of life in its diversity, richness, glory and tragedy, then it does so with reference to life defined by death. This is why spirituality should occupy such a prominent place in palliative care, but it is also why spirituality must also be more than a token. For some, spirituality is a relief and detachment from the struggles of existence; others may find through spirituality an affirmation or transfiguration of life in spite of death. This apparently paradoxical stance is nothing more than the reality of existence in its wholeness, which spirituality stands in symbolic relationship to. That language is often inadequate to render the spiritual dimension is evident. Conceptual and abstract words cannot convey the depth of spiritual experience just as the experience of music cannot be adequately described in documented accounts. But spirituality does not need to be abandoned to some ephemeral place appreciated by the gnostics. As with music, spirituality can also be coherently ordered, notated, discussed and developed.

Pursuing spirituality beyond its apprehensibility is a relevant discipline, therefore, for palliative care to be engaged with and, as importantly, to contribute to. Indeed, spirituality is a creative paradigm that should benefit from the wide range of contributors that we have been considering. It is perhaps, therefore, disappointing to discover how limited the involvement of palliative care has been so far. Of equal concern is the occlusion of spirituality from accounts of human experience and from the practice of health care. This is less a result of the abeyance of the spiritual and more a consequence of the loss of confidence in 'caring' professions to engage with this deeply human perspective of self and the world. The neglect or negation of spirituality within a particular field results in obscuration within

that field; but, as we explore in the next chapter, spirituality finds alternative expressions and places of validation, or creates new ones.

This chapter began by describing spirituality as something of a conundrum in palliative care. Conundrums become boring after a while, especially
when no solution is forthcoming, and thus become neglected or the object
of only occasional curiosity. The conundrum challenges palliative care to
engage seriously with spirituality and to afford it the same concern as other
domains. If spirituality has a place in palliative care, as its philosophy
suggests, it should not be treated lightly or dealt with in a cursory fashion.
More than that, the challenge is a far broader one concerning how we
understand well-being, suffering, life and death: and that is a matter which
none of us can avoid, and which shapes our own lives and our relationship
with others.

For those for whom the soul is an empty symbol, and spirituality a
remnant of a metaphysical world superseded by a plainly physical one, the
challenge may still find echoes in moral debates, the impact of suffering, the
questions of existence and the contemplation of mortality. The spiritual
side of life is a dynamic force that is not only deeply embedded in our
thoughts and ideas, but also experienced in our being human. It is this
persistent presence which requires addressing both individually and collectively and which constantly challenges our language, symbols and notions.
Understanding spirituality is, therefore, a rational intellectual activity, a
creative act involving the imagination, a contemplative exercise and a means
of grasping the quintessence of life.

> Maybe our mind should be sensitive to the vastness that lies behind all
> reality, should be open to the winds and whispers of infinity, and
> should be able – by inkling and intuition – to enter the hidden realms
> of the blazing Tyger, the Robin, the Eagle, the Unicorn, and our mys-
> terious humanity. How can we, in the presence of irreducible being,
> view life from only one perspective . . . ?
>
> (Okri 1997: 19–20)

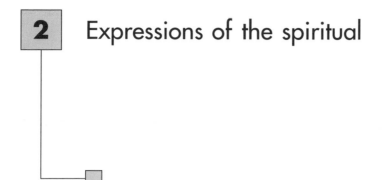

2 Expressions of the spiritual

The spiritual does not exist in the abstract, it is part of the lived experience of people. It therefore finds expression in the beliefs that people hold, their world-view, commitments, values and their individual and collective behaviour. Expressions of the spiritual are manifold, from highly regulated and patterned forms to fragmentary and disorganized types. People range across this spectrum and articulate the spiritual through traditional and institutional schemes, through newly established forms and through individualistic self-expression. The spectrum also extends in another plane, that ranging from the orthodox to the heterodox (or heretical depending upon your perspective). Orthodox manifestations of the spiritual conform to established definitions and teachings, often expounded through leaders and 'schools' reproduced in canonical 'texts'. The heterodox forms may be hybrids, relate loosely to established types and with less reference to accepted authorities and conventions. This rich diversity raises further questions about whether we can describe spirituality as a unitary concept, something that has a utility of convenience – a useful shorthand – but which has a severely reduced capacity for conveying subtlety and detail.

It is in the experience and expression of spirituality that definition is restored to bland profiles. But what are we to count as spiritual, how are we to differentiate it from other phenomena and what are its attributes? It may be of some help in this respect to consider spirituality something like an iceberg, with its visible portion belying a substantial submerged mass. The visible aspect of spirituality may represent only a limited part of something more extensive that has an internal aspect which is not directly visible. Behaviour, rituals, texts, symbols and customs may be considered some of the visible dimensions of spirituality. Perceptions, feelings, inchoate or unarticulated beliefs and thoughts may be some of the invisible dimensions which concern experiences of the transcendent, transcendental, numinous and sacred. It is the invisible dimensions that seldom register on surveys but which can be the most significant aspect for an individual and may underlie social expressions or co-exist in some unconnected way (Hay 1982). Despite a growth in interest in spirituality, many people maintain a reticence in discussing it or declaring what it means for them. This reluctance to disclose may be explained by a common view that it is something not talked about openly, it is a private matter. Equally, other professional, personal and social factors may contribute to constraints upon expressing spirituality.

The presence of spirituality in the empirical world is a matter that is intruding into the articles of health journals as much as it is reviving the interest of sociologists. What has been to a great extent hidden, discounted or ignored, save for few exceptions, is now emerging in paradigms and concepts, education syllabuses and conferences. Whether or not this can be explained as a rediscovery or as an attempt to address an insufficiency is an issue that runs through this book. And while many of these examples are observational, they do point to expressions of the spiritual that seem remarkably alive in the light of a predicted demise and death. Perhaps, then, spirituality has been buried, both by its very nature and more recently by the postmodern and secular theses. As we shall see in this chapter, what can be considered traditional forms of spirituality persist, but alongside them there are also new shoots appearing of a detraditionalized form, some of which are blossoming in the fertile soil of palliative care.

Religion

People whose spirituality is patterned around an organized system of beliefs collectively expressed in institutions, rituals and places may be considered to have a religious spirituality. Religions embody certain beliefs, ideals often represented in texts, symbols and practices, which refer to the sacred, transcendent and ultimate. It is a remarkably prevalent and dynamic human trait that is manifest in a vast array of belief systems, institutions and practices. At a basic level, religion can be understood as systems of knowledge orientated towards an ultimate goal, validated by their adherents and evolved through successive generations. The existence of so many religions raises the uncomfortable questions of logical incompatibility and truth, but it is also a reminder of humankind's compelling exploration for what it can become:

> It may be the case that religions are entirely wrong, or even just partly wrong, about what they believe to be the ultimate case; but that does not affect the point. The point is that what are on offer in religious

Figure 2.1 Dimensions of religion

Ritual/practical
Doctrinal/philosophical
Mythic/narrative
Experiential/emotional
Ethical/legal
Organizational/social
Material/artistic

Source: Smart 1996: 10–11

traditions are both the goals to which any humans may reasonably and hopefully aspire, and also the resources to help them make the journey.
(Bowker 1987: 11–12)

The goals of many religions are not focused beyond death, but concern life here and now, the way it is lived, celebrated, ennobled, forgiven and re-deemed. This is one reason why religion is such a major feature of human history and continues to play a significant role in the lives of many people, particularly when considered on a global scale. The apprehension of the sacred or holy, the sense of the numinous, the mystical or contemplative experience, are all realities for believers that shape ritual, motivate beha-viour and inspire faith and practice. It is tempting, therefore, to see such experiences as a lowest common denominator; but when considered within a particular social context and interpreted through a religious tradition, the case for a generic phenomenon becomes weaker. Human experience is as obviously diverse as it is similar, and religions differ in the way they are organized as systems, their anthropology, cosmology, rituals, resources, values, myths and world-view. However, it does not follow that we cannot use a sensitive pattern of fields with which to frame the foci of religions. Thus Smart (1989) suggests seven dimensions of religion which provide a balanced perspective and a means to describe a religion in functional terms (Figure 2.1). They counterbalance tendencies to view religions in mono-chrome by separating out distinct but interrelated phenomena.

The empirical presence of religion is unavoidable and so is its impression upon the ways in which people face illness, suffering and death. Religious narratives can impart meaning and significance to events which may other-wise be cast in more problematic or banal terms. Myths may contain ethical and doctrinal illustrations and implications that can be enacted and rein-forced through rituals. As rituals make external what is felt, believed and hoped for, so religions also find an external form reflected in the objects and icons of faith, specific places, artefacts and art. Finally, religions involve people in ways that are expressed through incorporation, society, cultures and politics. Thus religion finds its place in the law, ethics, the welfare state, the National Health Service and the philosophy of palliative care. It should also be recognized that palliative care is itself expressive of a world-view through which terminal illness, suffering and death are interpreted and responded to. The hospice tradition is in many ways a product of religion with its strong historical relationship to Christianity. This has been attenuated in palliative care where a more pluralistic and humanistic thanatology has been developed in a context of a National Health Service (Small 1998).

The fact of religion's existence in contemporary society (and a robust existence in some contexts) is in itself a fascinating and a confounding phenomenon when considered in the light of its many critics. It has been understood as both a symptom and a determinant of an 'anxious' society; an implausible world-view against 'rationalistic' certainties and the abandonment of metaphysics; an illusion; and, as Marx and Engels conceived it, an:

> ideology, false consciousness, the narcotic displacement activity of a soulless world, a form of vicarious happiness, of *bonheur*, within a socioeconomic framework that generates dissatisfaction and unhappiness and whose meaning and truth are sought and found in the class struggle and property relations.
>
> (Trías 1998: 97)

Religion, or approximations to it, interrogated by 'reason' come out badly because, like the humanity with which it is bound, it is explained in part through subjective experience, paradox and mystery. Critiques of religion do not eradicate finitude, pain, a sense of belonging, of the numinous, or transcendence. Nor do they eliminate emotional and instinctual urges to name God, to articulate belief and to live beyond reason among others who are committed to more than an empirical space. This is not to dismiss the important questions about the claims of religion, but it is to reiterate that religions are not in essence hypotheses. A religion, as Smart suggests in the use of seven dimensions, is a world-view manifest in diverse patterns involving the lived experiences, beliefs and behaviour of people.

Thrower (1999) points to the paradox that we are a generation that has never before had so much knowledge of religion and yet we are the least religious of people. However, the amount of knowledge we now possess about religion hinders our explanations of religion and mitigates against a grand all-encompassing theory. Thrower suggests that there are two broad categories of theories advanced to explain religion: the religious and the naturalistic, in other words those that accept the transcendental claims of religion and those which explain religion through a human discourse

Table 2.1   Theories of religion

Religious theories	Naturalistic theories
Revelation	Human construct
Experience	Primitive error
Philosophy	Psychological construct
	Social construct

Source: Thrower 1999

(Table 2.1). What is apparent is that these theories represent distinctive cultures and some of the leading intellectual figures of the past:

> These range from the claim that religion is a response to the revealed word of God (Judaism, Christianity and Islam), that it is a way of life founded on 'the word' heard by the sage of old showing the way to final release from the eternal round of birth and rebirth (Hinduism and, in a qualified way, Buddhism), that it is the path to the existential realisation of the soul's identity with God or to union with God or Ultimate Reality (a variety of Indian and Western thinkers), to the claim that it is a primitive and now outmoded way of seeking to explain, predict and control events in the world (Tylor, Frazer and, in a qualified way, Horton), a roundabout way in which human beings have talked about themselves (Feuerbach and, in a qualified way, Berger), the fantastic realisation of the human essence in a world where the human essence has no true reality and an ideology legitimating the status quo (Marx), the revenge of the weak on the strong (Nietzsche), a regression to an infantile trust in a 'father-figure' in the face of the harsh realities of the world (Freud), a societies' celebration of itself (Durkheim), or a way of reconciling human beings to their fate (Weber and Malinowski).
>
> (Thrower 1999: 202)

The personal aspect of religion is one that is often the focus of palliative care, both in terms of service provision and in its effect upon a person's approach to illness, dying and death. It is in the individual that we find the interaction between the personal, the social and the cultural, where beliefs, participation and experience interrelate. This is also the context in which many hypotheses have been suggested for why religion exists and continues to operate in the lives of so many. Beit-Hallahmi and Argyle (1997) provide a useful summary of the main psychological explanations of religion which they group into three categories: origin hypotheses which account for the psychological sources of religion; maintenance hypotheses which explain

Table 2.2   Psychological explanations of religion

Origin hypotheses	Maintenance hypotheses	Consequence hypotheses
Neural factors	Social learning	Personal integration
Cognitive need	Identity and self-esteem	Social integration
Cognitive styles:	Deprivation explanations	
evolutionary optimism	Personality factors	
religion as art		
Adjustment to anxiety		
Fear of death		
The effects of early		
childhood		
Projections and religious		
beliefs		
Super-ego projection and		
guilt		
Sexual motivation		

Source: Beit-Hallahmi and Argyle 1997: 11

why people hold religious beliefs; and consequence hypotheses which concern the effects of religion upon individuals and society (see Table 2.2).

The human search for meaning, existential insecurity, the transmission of beliefs and behaviour through culture, and the need for a unifying value system are some of the many reasons why a person may be religious. However, psychology's search for cause and effect – the stimuli and consequences of religion – can never do justice to the biographical accounts of the people we meet, for whom religion is more than theory. A poignant example of this was given by the playwright Dennis Potter, whose wrestling with religion was expressed in his plays and in an interview he gave a few weeks before he died from cancer. In the interview, Potter dismisses the compensatory reasons for religion (which address fear and provide hope) and affirms an intuition and assumption of God's presence:

Religion has always been – I've said it before, it doesn't matter that I repeat myself, I won't get many more chances to repeat myself, thank God – but religion to me has always been the wound, not the bandage. I don't see the point of not acknowledging the pain and misery and the grief of the world, and if you say, 'Ah but God understands' or 'Through that you come to a greater appreciation' . . . I mean, I don't think, well you nasty old sod, if that's God . . . that's no God, that's not my God, that's not how I see God. I see God in us or with us, if I see at all, as some shreds and particles and rumours, some knowledge that we have, some feeling why we sing and dance and act, why we paint, why we love, why we make art. All the things that separate us from the purely animal in us are palpably there, and you can call them what you like, and you can theologize about them and you can build great structures of belief about them. The fact is they are there and I have no means of knowing whether that thereness in some sense doesn't cling to what I call me.

(Potter 1994: 5–6)

In Britain, most people express a Christian nominalism, in other words they have a low religiosity but retain beliefs to some extent. Davie (1994) calls this the 'common religion' of individuals, set within a society permeated with Christianity in its various dimensions, but where 'believing without belonging' is a persistent pattern. However, it would be a mistake to polarize people into those, for example, who practise a religious faith and those who just believe. There is a far greater spread in people's beliefs and practices than allowed for in a discrete account. Religion, as we have noted, is a multidimensional variable and many factors contribute to the particular form and content of religion with which a person identifies. The interlocking relationship of the dimensions of religion can be seen if we take the idea of religious worship:

The practice of worship supposes a superior, indeed awe-inspiring, personal Being (or Beings). So the practice implies a doctrine. But the doctrine itself, in supposing a *personal* Being . . . also supposes a Being about whom stories or narratives can be said: in short such a Being has a mythic dimension. And so in talking of worship we speak of something about whom or which three dimensions come into play.

(Smart 1996: 70)

It is not difficult to expand a consideration of worship to seven dimensions. The point is that approaching religion from one aspect can lead into others. It also suggests how a sensitive understanding of religion may reveal an often neglected but rich 'picture' of a person's world-view. None of this requires that an enquirer should hold that the beliefs are valid, experiences plausible or worship meaningful, but it does require a respect for a person's world-view and its 'reality'. The patient who has had an overwhelming sense of peace and believes it to be a sign of God's presence, or the patient who has railed against God is expressing many more things than just theology. A professional attending the patient may not share a belief in a God of this nature but can appreciate why it matters to the patient.

A more difficult issue concerns the question of conflicting world-views between professionals, patients and carers. Leaving aside ethical and legal duties of professionals, it is helpful to realize how the dimensions of a religion operate in a person's life and where behaviour and choices are contingent upon beliefs. This may not always be articulated with singular clarity because beliefs are enmeshed and incorporated into a person's way of life. However, a discerning professional, aware of a person's religious orientation and its meaning to the person, should at least be able explore more fundamental reasons for decisions and requests.

It has been noted tentatively above that the common religion of British people is Christian nominalism, but as we have seen, religion is far more complex and subtle than a convenient label suggests. We are also well aware in England of considerable religious diversity in the midst of a nation which has an established faith, namely Christianity in the form of Anglicanism. Trying to give detail to this terrain is a task fraught with dangers and difficulties. Many of the dangers occur in attempting comparisons and in the search for reliable evidence, with difficulties in interpreting data and sometimes in providing basic definitions. Bauman offers us a cautionary but helpful insight from a 'postmodern' perspective:

> 'Religion' belongs to the family of curious, and often embarrassing concepts, which one perfectly understands until one wants to define them. Postmodern mind, for once, agrees to issue this family, mal-treated or sentenced to deportation by the modern scientific reason, with a permanent residence permit. Postmodern mind, more tolerant (since better aware of its own weakness) than its modern predecessor and critic, resigns itself to the tendency of definitions to conceal as much as they reveal and to maim and obfuscate while pretending to clarify and straighten up. It also accepts the fact that all too often experience spills out of the verbal cages in which one would wish to hold it, that there are things of which one should keep silent since one cannot speak of them, and that the ineffable is as much an integral part of the human mode of being-in-the world as is the linguistic net in which one tries (in vain, as it happens, though no less vigorously for that reason) to catch it.
>
> (Bauman 1998: 55)

Proceeding with caution, and aware of the problems of presenting a re-stricted view, what is the religious terrain that palliative care looks out onto and whose constituents it cares for? The Multi-faith Directory Research Project offers sensitive estimates of some community figures which attempt to steer a course between speculative statistics, data extrapolated from the 1991 census and sample studies, and figures taken from the records and research of specific communities. These are put alongside figures of active members that are given in the *UK Christian Handbook: Religious Trends* which are formed from estimates and other sources depending upon how a religion defines and records membership as well as similar extrapolations (see Table 2.3).

The figures in the table are highly sensitive, not necessarily consistent, and able to withstand comparison of a minimal nature. The two columns

Table 2.3   UK religious membership figures 1995

	Community membership	Active membership
Baháis	6000	6000
Buddhists	30,000–130,000	45,000
Christians	40,000,000	6,361,318
Hindus	400,000–550,000	155,000
Jains	25,000–30,000	10,000
Jews	300,000	93,684
Muslims	1,000,000–1,500,000	580,000
Sikhs	350,000–500,000	350,000
Zoroastrians	5000–10,000	2500

Source: adapted from Weller (1997: 30) and *UK Christian Handbook Religious Trends No.1* (1998–99 ed), Brierley (1997: 2.6, 10.12–10.15)

show something of the disparity between active membership and 'those who in some way identify with a particular religious tradition, including children and adults, *whether or not* they are actively involved in any organization within the religion concerned' (Weller 1997: 30). The figures offer no distinction between different schools, denominations and traditions within many of the religions, and they aggregate regional and local variations.

To each person included in these figures could be put a mass of additional questions concerning the strength of their beliefs, the extent to which they practise them, their involvement in the community and ritual life of the religion, their moral attitudes and their experiences. Little of this information is available in any extensive or reliable form. Bold statistics reflect crude representations and provoke many questions that usually have to remain unanswered owing to lack of supporting information and associated data. In addition, these are figures of reasonably large communities; an expanding number of smaller religious groups and new religious movements could be added to them.

When there is the opportunity to explore some of the strata underlying the religious terrain, more variables come into play and more variations can be discerned. The British Social Attitudes survey of 1995 (reported in Brierley 1997) questioned people about their belief in God according to six responses (Table 2.4). The figures reflect a spectrum of belief from what could be classed as a clear theism to a clear atheism. However, the inclusion of additional variables reflects the significance of age and gender, suggesting both a generational difference as well as a consistent theme that women are more religious than men (Davie 1994: ch. 7).

The diversity of religions among the potential patients of palliative care has raised the issue of what provisions there are in a service to meet specific needs. The National Council for Hospice and Specialist Palliative Care

Table 2.4   People's belief in God

	Total %	% under 35	% 35–54	% 55 or over	% men	% women
I know God really exists and I have no doubt about it	23	13	22	35	18	27
While I have doubts, I feel I do believe in God	24	21	28	24	20	28
I find myself believing in God some of the time, but not at others	13	11	14	12	10	15
I don't believe in a personal God, but I do believe in a Higher Power of some kind	13	15	14	8	15	11
I don't know whether there is a God, and I don't believe there is any way to find out	16	23	12	15	21	12
I don't believe in God	11	17	10	6	16	7

Source: adapted from Brierley (1997: 5.13)

Services has considered, for example, how accessible services are for black and ethnic minority people and asked whether the 'perceived environment' of a unit may alienate people (Hill and Penso 1997). Religion, culture and ethnicity are often treated in such discussion as more-or-less similar and make use of categories and classifications to convey easily the prescribed needs of black and ethnic minority people. Information about different groups is often perceived to be the solution to deficits in a service in order that professionals will know what to do or know whom to call. But such cultural and religious scripts tend to contain objective accounts of social practices and the need for specific facilities, food and artefacts which can pre-empt professionals exploring the subjective needs and experience of individuals. It has also been argued that, whilst comforting to professionals, crude multicultural approaches do little to remove barriers and can legitimize discrimination (Gunaratnam 1997). This approach can also fail to account for demographic and epidemiological factors when analysing why some groups appear to be underrepresented in the patient population. It is generally silent about people from communities which do not register in the limited categories available.

Religion in palliative care is often dealt with in a checklist and responded to according to policy and sequestered as a matter of a personal nature between a patient and the appropriate religious representative. Attitudes of intolerance, disrespect and discomfort reinforce the obscurity and reductionism of religion, limit research into this field and may hinder open and sensitive discussions between patients, carers and professionals. Rather than treating religion as an optional adjunct, its prevalent role needs recognizing both as an aspect of the illness narrative and for its potential therapeutic benefits (Dein and Stygall 1997). But an important counter-argument stands in the way of this approach and requires consideration, and that is the argument that religion is an increasingly inconsequential aspect of contemporary society. This is an argument which cannot be limited to religion, but ranges across the breadth of spirituality.

Sacred and secular

To the God of absence and of aftermath, .
of the anchor in the sea, the brimming sea . . .
whose truant omnipresence sets us free
from this world, and firmly on the one true path,
with our cup of shadows overflowing, with
our hearts uplifted, heavy and half-starved,
let us honour Him who made the Void, and carved
these few words from the thin air of our faith.

(Paterson 1999: 43)

Secular is used commonly to denote something that has nothing to do with religion or the sacred. It relates to the civil as opposed to the ecclesiastical and refers to a worldly as opposed to spiritual perspective. Qualifying a subject as secular is an attempt to denote the absence of religious influence and the presence of rationalistic and humanistic values, ideas and practice, hence a 'secular funeral'. Thus secularization can be understood as a process of the reorientation of society around non-religious norms.

Explanations for this reorientation away from religion are substantially premised upon the transition to a modern way of life. This has brought about profound transformations, over three centuries, that have gradually and comprehensively altered our modes of life and our concept of the world. It is claimed that there are many contributing factors involved in this shift. One element provides an example of the secular argument. Knowledge, understanding and practice are examined and revised in the light of empirical science. This becomes a circular process of reflection, interpretation and application, in which knowledge is corrigible, waiting for revision, and this tends towards discontinuity and instability. Reflexivity, theories suggest, is a process which can question continuity and contradict historical experience. The tenets of religion thus become eroded and the certainties provided by tradition can become archaic. When combined with other conditions, modernity is inherently secularizing, and although the result is not a complete loss of religion, Giddens argues that:

> most of the situations of modern social life are manifestly incompatible with religion as a pervasive influence upon day-to-day life. Religious cosmology is supplanted by reflexively organised knowledge, governed by empirical observation and logical thought, and focussed upon material technology and socially applied codes. Religion and tradition were always closely linked, and the latter is even more thoroughly undermined than the former by the reflexivity of modern social life, which stands in direct opposition to it.
>
> (Giddens 1990: 109)

Modernization, according to this thesis, is a mode of social life that creates an adverse environment for religion and where it is generally no longer required or involved. Bruce (1996) adduces three salient features of the structure of modern society that result in secularization. The first is the fragmentation of life into particular areas and domains so that where there was once commonality and an overarching shape to life, now there is stratification and separation. Religion becomes a special and optional area rather than a widespread aspect of life. The second feature concerns a shift from the communal to the societal locus of life. This opens up possibilities for pluralism and weakens cohesive values and beliefs. It also relocates people from a community in which they belong to a society in which they are relatively anonymous and where beliefs become personal. Thirdly, religion in the face of rationality becomes less plausible, its explanations of life are challenged by scientific explanations, and its scope for influence is limited by the expansion of technology and its control of the natural world. Taken together, the consequence for religion is that it loses its impact and its place in society, and for the individual therefore it loses its purchase in shaping a common coherent orientation:

> individual beliefs which are not regularly articulated and affirmed in a group, which are not refined and burnished by shared ceremonies, which are not the object of regular and systematic elaboration, and which are not taught to the next generation or to outsiders are unlikely to exert much influence on the actions of those who hold them and are even less likely to have significant social consequences.
>
> (Bruce 1996: 58–9)

Secularization does not spell a bright future for religion in its traditional form as the conclusion is its inevitable dysfunction. However, when considered as a phenomenon rather than just a function, religion contradicts some of the most sceptical analyses and limits secularism. Factors which were once cited as key reasons for religion's demise have themselves declined in their significance and others have contributed to fostering religion. Industrialization is no longer a dominant theme for many western countries, but moral and existential questions arise with new medical technology. Countervailing movements have also appeared which have sought unitary concepts amidst difference, such as the idea of a common humanity with universal rights or religious diversity within a single spiritual frame. The differences of modernity can consequently become transparent to commonality and the secular can become the place of the sacred.

Religion in contemporary society is evidently present in manifold ways and contradicts the polarizing prognosis of secularization. When considered in cultural terms, religion 'is highly flexible and unpredictable, appearing in a plethora of guises and forms with a variety of consequences. It may seek to conserve but, equally, to challenge or to change' (Lyon 1996: 23). Few arguments for secularization take account of the dynamic and dialectic nature of religion and so portray a progressive society leaving behind a static outmoded and dysfunctional religion. The vestige of religion that survives in the world of the secularist is little more than a heritage. But the dimensions of religion present in contemporary society are more prevalent, diverse and active than this suggests. Perhaps what is more evident is that organized religion and its institutions have become largely abstracted from significant social roles (for example, education and health care) such that religion and society intersect in fewer places. In other words the context of religion has changed alongside the infrastructure of social life, human thought and experience. Religion is a matter of choice in many societies rather than the accepted common world-view, it exists in a pluralistic situation and becomes part of a synthesis of manifold beliefs. Therefore if we consider the functions of religion in the societies of north-west Europe, Smart suggests that:

> there is a much wider worldview or set of values to which people adhere, and within that a small part is played by traditional religion, as a kind of solemn ornament at crucial passages in a person's life and in the life of the community ... But this wider worldview goes beyond the older standpoint of faith. Values are not subordinated to an overarching religious cosmology and philosophy, but religion tends to be fitted in a complex metaphysics which embodies prominent ideas from science, views about how to run the state and values derived from the media and elsewhere.
>
> (Smart 1996: 262)

Religion is not so much sequestrated but repositioned (or abandoned) alongside other 'reality-defining agencies' (Berger 1967: 127) thus dispersing its efficacy and challenging its plausibility and legitimacy. In palliative care, religion is generally recognized as a resource for patients, operating in a carefully defined way, often in the form of a chaplain and a chapel. In some instances religion provides the emblem for the organization and represents something of the value-base of the service philosophy. The legitimacy of religion in palliative care is derived in part from the high respect for patient autonomy, which may include a need for religious expression and ministry. Its plausibility derives in particular from its ability to work close to the edge of life and at death where few others have as much to offer in terms of ritual. This is reinforced by the common use of clergy to conduct funerals, although a major shift from burial to cremation, especially since 1945, marks a change in both theology and customary practice (Davies 1990).

It is difficult in the UK to avoid aspects of the sacred and dimensions of religion which are embedded into the culture, however dormant these may be for many of the people for much of the time. But traditional religion has lost a considerable proportion of its critical social mass so that the environment has become open to different forms of religious expression which seek to offer a fulfilling alternative. Prominent among them, although already to some extent diffused within the wider religious terrain, is a form of contemporary spirituality that is apparently disassociated from traditional religion and which has found some assimilation within the practices and beliefs of palliative care.

Spirituality of a new age

A discourse of spirituality whose locus is the individual 'self' predicates the New Age movement which has influenced not only religion but also ideas and practices concerned with healing and well-being. There is no orthodox form of New Age religion, but some of its common themes (for example, human potential, environmentalism, esoteric knowledge and reincarnation) have achieved a certain popularity and acceptance. As with other forms of religion, there are levels of involvement and belief to which people are committed, but New Age differs from most others in its scope and in its toleration of diversity. This eclecticism is part of its appeal, for it 'means that there are few clear divisions and boundaries, few organizations, but rather a milieu in which people acquire, absorb, and learn a variety of beliefs and practices that they combine into their own pockets of culture' (Bruce 1996: 200).

The New Age provides us with an emblematic paradigm of religion in contemporary culture that to some extent epitomizes the interrelated social processes so far discussed. According to Lyon, the New Age relates in some ways to the so-called postmodern condition in that it is mobilized in response to the spiritual vacuum of modernity, 'centering on the self, being undogmatic, involving networks rather than an institutional base' (Lyon 1996: 21). These broad characteristics suggest a spirituality whose primary reference is the subject rather than any institution or empirical reality. It is one which is often centred around expressions of self rather than the numinous and resembles a form of self-build system of beliefs, values and practices that engages with an eclectic mix of religious and philosophical ideas. It is what is within the individual that matters, the experience of which provides the source of authority, wisdom and spirituality. In his authoritative writing on the subject, Heelas presents a useful overall picture:

> New Agers see the person divided into that which belongs to artifices of society and culture and that which belongs to the depths of human nature. Inspired by spiritual disciplines or practices rather than by dogmas, beliefs or codified moralities, participants become aware of what they *are* . . . More comprehensively, the New Age is a highly optimistic, celebratory, utopian and spiritual form of humanism, many versions . . . also emphasizing the spirituality of the natural order as a whole. Ultimacy – God, the Goddess, the Higher Self – lies within, serving as the source of vitality, creativity, love, tranquillity, wisdom, responsibility, power and all those other qualities which are held to comprise the perfect inner life and which, when applied in daily practice (supposedly) ensure that all is utopian.
>
> (Heelas 1996: 28)

The utopian appeal of New Age has parallels in other forms of religion in which salvation depends upon divinity, but in a religion of self it has only humanity. However, the appeal of New Age is broader than a path to perfection because it provides a way of coping with modernity. Dissatisfaction with a contemporary way of life that fails to satisfy may be part of what prompts some people to seek an alternative or replacement approach. Paradoxically, according to Heelas, the New Age also appeals because it exemplifies aspects of modernity, such as the autonomy of the individual, and provides 'solutions' by a radical extension of particular familiar cultural values, such as the notion of the 'sacred' nature of humanity. Taken together, along with many other factors, it is a religion without a traditional system of beliefs or social institution:

> Crudely, detraditionalized people want detraditionalized religion: a 'religion' which is (apparently) more constructed than given; with practices which emphasize the authority of participants; which enables participants to be personally responsible for their salvation . . . which provides guidance and personal experience rather than beliefs; which does not demand that one should belong to a particular organization. This, then is a spirituality which (it appears) enables one to explore one's *own* innerSelf; which allows one the freedom to *be* oneSelf, which enables one to discover oneself, rather than handing the task over to others.
>
> (Heelas 1996: 172–3)

If we consider the primacy of a spiritual self in New Age to be a consequence of modernity, then the centrality of the individual patient can be
considered as an approximate analogy in palliative care. In crude terms
these can be understood as consequences of contemporary society and the
processes that form it. Religion is within this process even though its sacred
dimension may be premised upon eternal truths and a belief in divinity
beyond the flux of the world. There are other approximate analogies that
can be drawn between these two movements: a utopian vision (in palliative
care the 'good death'), a philosophy of holism and its 'universal' spiritual
dimension, a critique of allopathic medicine and the acceptance of alternative therapies, the significance of personal experience, self-exploration
and self-expression. Both movements have come to fruition in a period of
social transition in which western scientific medicine has been subject to
accusations of scientism, social monopoly, ineffectiveness and financial
determinism. The biomedical model has failed totally to convince a growing
number of people in a populace in which:

> Affluence, education, leisure and many of the values promoted by cor-
> porate capitalism have stoked a culture of individual enhancement and
> free and active choice. As with cars, careers or sexual partners, it
> has become the done thing to shop around for healing – whether in
> desperation, as an exercise of the power of the purse, or as part of
> an odyssey of life . . . Flexibility, permissiveness, variety, self-discovery
> have assumed greater status in our culture of self-enhancement or
> narcissism. There is a new self-assertiveness among the sick, perhaps a
> survival strategy in the teeth of extreme depersonalization and
> bureaucratization of regular medicine.
>
> (Porter 1997: 689)

There are many factors that provided the impetus and opportunity for the
development of the modern hospice movement and palliative care, but to
borrow Heelas's observation, it is an ideal that provides both an alternative
as well as radical interpretation of the conventional. The point, however, is
not any implied correlation between the two movements but their response
to similar concerns. This has promoted the acceptance of contemporary
forms of religion and spirituality as an integral component of palliative care
as well as a demonstration of its philosophy. It is of particular interest that
some of the complementary or alternative therapies which have become a
feature of many palliative care services often have an affinity with New Age
science and healing practices. In addition, the significance of the patient's
narrative, the promotion of the patient's quest for meaning, and quality of
life are all themes of palliative care that have religious counterparts.

In concluding this chapter of complex themes and issues we are reminded
that many expressions of the spiritual are closely related to religion even
when these expressions are detraditionalized. Religion remains 'within our

horizon and challenges us to think its truth' (Trías 1998: 102), and its influence can still be clearly traced within palliative care. However, shifts in society have impacted upon the religious climate to the extent that a wide range of beliefs and practices are tolerated and available for individuals to choose among. This includes new religious forms, although how innovative they are remains debatable. Contemporary expressions of the spiritual permeate palliative care in the philosophies of personhood, well-being, dying and death which it absorbs from the cultural context in which it is embedded. Palliative care also opens its doors to complementary therapies and beliefs which reflect diverse understandings of the sacred. That these spiritual expressions exist is not remarkable in itself, but that they seldom become the subject of enquiry or dialogue is notable because it may suggest that palliative care fails to understand spirituality beyond the individual level where even there it is often restricted to religious activity. In doing so it fails to recognize how the spiritual dimension relates to people's worldviews and how this is manifested in the wider contexts of organizations and society. This is no more apparent than in the matter of death, and it is this that we consider in the next chapter.

3 Dying and death: a spiritual place?

Dying has traditionally been the territory of the spiritual *par excellence*. Here was the place where, in the Middle Ages, the final rite of passage required preparation, assistance and ritual to ensure the soul's salvation. The 'art of dying' was a process that involved the living in keeping vigil and administering last rites, and it involved the dying person in the supernatural battle that ensued around the bedside between the angelic hosts and the demonic hordes. The moment of death was the moment of destiny when God released the soul to its fate (Muir 1997). The living were expected to prepare for their demise with devotional exercises and were daily reminded of their mortality by common visual artefacts and texts. Foremost among these was the moralistic 'dance of death' which portrayed the inescapable and indiscriminate nature of death (Llewellyn 1991). Until the present century there was little to stand in the way of death, but today the dance of death has become subject to different choreography:

> The patient suffers, the family threatens, the colleagues frown, the nurse laughs, Death grins, and the young doctor dances a crazy jig amidst the tumult, while once he dreamt he would glide along the floor with Death in a perfectly controlled tango.
>
> (Keizer 1997: 30)

Modern medicine developed the power to wrestle with death and attempted to control it with sometimes desperate efforts to maintain somatic life. But at a time when medical advances generated considerable expectations in the ability of doctors to cure and prevent death, people with terminal malignant disease were often denied their diagnosis, afforded poor symptom control and left to die in isolated hospital rooms. Death was a sign of failure in a predominantly curative system; it had become depersonalized, desacralized and a terminal clinical event. It was this type of grim experience, both of the dying and those who witnessed their deaths, that provided a major impetus for the development of the modern hospice movement which has attempted to reaffirm a spiritual aspect of dying and death.

Death is at the margin of life and yet occupies much of its central features. There is an enormous amount of human thought, behaviour, art, religion, finance, science and technology devoted to death: its causes, its purpose, its timing, its place, its consequences and its endless intractable mysteries. Death sets the limit of life, and through this antithesis defines so much of what it means to live, of what it is to be human. Therefore the diagonal of mortal existence, of being and non-being, raises questions about the significance of living and dying and remains *the* permanent existential challenge. Finally, death imposes loss through absence, punctuates familiar continuity with irreversible change, incites severe emotions and presents an unwanted demand to say farewell. In a consequential sense, death happens to the living who have to deal with the dead and who come to interpret it, make meaning out of it, find purpose in it, declare it through ritual and garland it with myth.

Death is fundamental to life, it is a critical determinant of human existence, and it bears a profound significance because it marks the end of what we value as intrinsically precious. This is an important reason why individual human life is understood as sacred because it is irreplaceable, it warrants not just respect and honour, but an absolute sense of sanctity too. This conviction of inviolability is rooted in beliefs about the uniqueness of humankind and in the idea that human life is the result of astonishing natural and human creation and investment. Death matters not just because of the oblivion or salvation it may signal, but also because it is the end of everything we have known and lived. This may explain why most people want their dying and the manner of their death to have some continuity and integrity with their lives (Dworkin 1993). The sacred nature of life finds an unequalled focus in its conclusion, which is why, for many people, dying and death are holy ground because of the intensity they bring to what is precious and meaningful.

He loved the sense of concentration, like the beam of light from a torch, focussed on this spot, the stillness and expectancy, the feeling that everything that had ever been in this one human life was packed now into the smallest space . . .

From the first time, he had felt its absolute importance to him, to sit in silence like this, watching for the tide to run, and been overwhelmed by the certainty that this small, uninteresting space, contained everything of significance. Within it, time shrank to a pinpoint, steadied and was still, the focus of the past, present and future, at the centre of the turning world.

(Hill 1998: 6–7)

Death has a significance beyond the cessation of the living, for in it we see what death could be like for ourselves, and by it we are reminded that the values, beliefs, commitments and hopes that we embody must have an end, even though they may persist in the lives of others. In this sense, death is as much about the future for the living as it is for the dead. But death is more than this, for it is also understood as the point of departure for the dying person which has posthumous consequences for the living and, for many, postmortem prospects for the dead. In considering the subject of death in this broad perspective it becomes more than the cancellation of embodied existence and suggests possibilities that transcend the physical boundaries.

Death is nothing

Death is significant both as a universal symbol of mortality and as a particular end to an individual life. It has also been accorded moral value, not least in the assertion by the hospice movement that the dying ought to attain a good death, or perhaps more accurately, a good dying, in which the values of personhood are maintained as far as possible. This concept depends upon the notion of the good life which stands in stark contrast to the death which negates it. However, the simple asymmetry between life and death – usually that life is good and death is bad – must be used carefully, because the two do not equate. There is no correspondence in death to the condition of being alive, there is only their absence because death is not an experiential state, and there is no person, in the general way that this is understood, to feel and know death. This suggests that death can be understood as nothing as it contains neither threat nor promise and that therefore mortality, rather than being significant, is just a matter of fact.

The opposing view to this is that mortality is humankind's greatest burden because it is the greatest threat. Death occupies a central place in the psychology of survival and in the behaviour that people adopt to avert this disaster. Death in this account becomes not a neutral object but one of fear and anxiety. It is the awareness that death is the inescapable negation of life which is the cause of insecurity because it is always present. Death, therefore, is the ultimate and absolute universal threat which forms the 'permanent horizon within which the anxiety of fate is at work' (Tillich 1952: 43). Life is incomparably better then death, or more accurately what is feared of death:

> Ay, but to die, and go we know not where;
> To lie in cold obstruction, and to rot;
> This sensible warm motion to become
> A kneaded clod; and the delighted spirit
> To bathe in fiery floods or to reside
> In thrilling region of thick-ribbed ice; . . .

The weariest and most loathed worldly life
That age, ache, penury, and imprisonment,
Can lay on nature is a paradise
To what we fear of death.

(*Measure for Measure*, III. i. 120–6, 130–3)

Death results in nothing in both these types of account, nothing meaning the end of existence, but to one this is of no concern while to the other it is of every concern. In both accounts death is destructive and an annihilation from which nothing can exist (Soll 1998). It is doubtful that this neat philosophical divide is reflected in how most people think of death. Equally, as we shall consider, it seems probable that the meaning of death for many people, and the attitude they hold towards it, is more complex and dynamic than these two accounts suggest. There is, however, another type of account which understands death as nothing because it is not the end, but a moment that points to an ultimate destiny, however this is conceived. Death is not complete destruction, something endures and is transformed, there is some form of survival. This is an understanding that finds popular representation in the words that Scott Holland, for example, gave to the face of death:

'Death is nothing at all. It does not count. I have only slipped away into the next room. Nothing has happened . . .' Nothing that we see in this dead material now laid out under our eyes represents or involves or includes the thing that was alive. That which we loved is not here. That is all. It has dropped out. It has slid away. We are as sure of this as we are of our own identity. We cannot conceive any other possibility. Reason and imagination alike repudiate it . . . All that matters shall go on as if death had never been.

(Scott Holland 1919: 126–7)

These are words of religious faith that see through death to a continued existence. In this account it is earthly life which is extinguished, and the nothing, the end of existence, is transcended. In most major world religions, 'life' is set within a cosmic panorama, with temporal life set against a horizon of eternity. Death thus becomes something which is both ending and beginning, through which there persists a continuity. Religions deal with death, and although the finality of death may be tempered by a post-mortem prospect, religious ritual, myth and doctrine take the fact of death and its impact on the living seriously, and certainly not as nothing.

Death is also seriously present in contemporary society where, for example, the media include its brutal details to illustrate news and where the extraordinary control of death is subject to popular representation and discourse. But to some extent the public spectacle and profile of death is in contrast to a general absence of death from public space (Mellor 1993). Death may be considered nothing for society in that it often takes place in professional spaces or is portrayed as an incident outside of the ordinary routine. Death is rarely paraded through the street but is dealt with discreetly outside of the city. Intimate death exists obscurely in a culture in which unknown death has high symbolic visibility and so the 'conventional' public death overshadows the presence of private death.

The intrusion of death into life is managed, explained and represented in a variety of approaches, some of which signify aspects of death as nothing. Death may be a terminus rather than a boundary crossed, and a terminus that for some may be better reached at speed. For those who believe in something beyond the end of life, death is a change of state and a transition. In the nothing of existence 'death is nothing' because either we cannot experience being dead or the end is also a beginning. Both provide a reason not to fear death. Death, however, is rarely a logic of nothing for the living because it figures in all our lives as the ending of our worldly future, our aspirations, our possibilities, our relationships. Solomon reminds us that, 'Being human – not just being philosophical – involves having some complex set of beliefs, expectations, hopes, worries and fears about death, death as death, death as disappearance, death as absence, death as frustration of ideals and desires' (Solomon 1998: 171). He also suggests that the fear of death is related not only to what the end signifies but also to the tangible prospect of what happens to the body, which does not become nothing, but the subject of decay, disposal and ritual. Lynch, a funeral director and poet, observes that:

> In a world where 'dysfunctional' has become the operative adjective, a body that has ceased to work has, it would seem, few useful applications – its dysfunction more manifest than the sexual and familial forms that fill our tabloids and talk shows. But a body that doesn't work is, in the early going, the evidence we have of a person who has ceased to be. And a person who has ceased to be is as compelling a prospect as it was when Neanderthal first dug holes for his dead, shaping the questions we still shape in the face of death: 'Is that all there is?, 'What does it mean?', 'Why is it cold?', 'Can it happen to me?'
> (Lynch 1998: 23–4)

The corpse, the most immediate consequence of death, is a significant body, demanding attention, emotions, care and ritual. It is the living that have to deal with death, their own and that of others, and it is the living for whom death is always something, even if that means contemplating absence and annihilation. This is a place, therefore, where people seek meanings in order to live with death, where death is interpreted through beliefs and where communities impose and enact meaning. It is also a place where people may encounter an aspect of the holy, in that death uniquely stops the mundane course of a life and imposes eternity, both in terms that it is absolute and unchanging (endless) as well as in the sense that it may translate the lost to the realm of the immortal (changeless). But, as we shall see, the sense of the holy may also be shaped by the customs and rituals with which we endow death.

Facing death

A person's comprehension of death and the meaning attributed to death will mediate death's impact. Beliefs and doctrines held about death will also play a part in the way that death is faced and attended to. Personal meanings will influence emotional reactions and shape the way that death is understood. To take just one example from a prolific literature on the subject, a sample of 265 American students aged 19 to 55 years of age enrolled in Death and Dying classes yielded three types of meaning: death as extinction, death as the beginning of an afterlife, and death as marking a legacy of life achievement. These were in turn correlated with the way in which death was perceived to be a threat or a danger in terms of both the dying process and the postmortem fate. This study showed that the meanings of death were differentially related to eight dimensions of the fear of death, including the fate of the body, pain, indignity and leaving loved ones (Cicirelli 1998: 713–33).

Attitudes to death will depend in part upon many variables such as experiences of death, cultural context, beliefs, religiosity, gender and age – factors not always accounted for in studies. Tomer and Eliason (1996) have proposed a comprehensive model regarding the concept of death anxiety which they take to mean 'a negative emotional reaction provoked by the anticipation of a state in which the self does not exist' (Tomer and Eliason 1996: 345). The three immediate determinants of death anxiety in this model stem from a person's self-awareness and contemplation of mortality. This activates a review of the past and a contemplation of the future that may induce regrets about unattained goals and unattainable aspirations. It also evokes an individual's beliefs about death and raises the question as to whether death makes any sense (see Figure 3.1). This process may be modified through the way a person copes with a heightened awareness of death and the concepts of self and the world in which this is situated. The person may therefore have a reduced death anxiety because of lack of regrets and a purposeful concept of death.

The model demonstrates consistency with some developmental psychological theories which posit that through self-actualization a person develops a lack of existential anxiety and a greater sense of transcendence, selflessness and relinquishment. It also accommodates a theme which is found in religious philosophies that suggest that it is only in realizing our momentary nature and by being ready for death that we can live fully, freed from fears and from efforts to avoid death. However, individuals may not be as consistent as a theoretical syntax suggests: attainments in life may not diminish

Figure 3.1   Tomer and Eliason's model of death anxiety

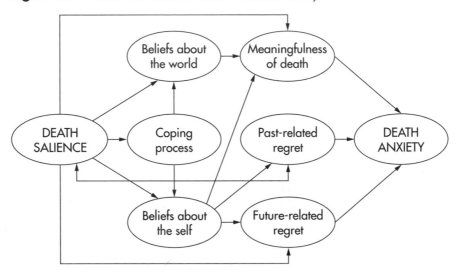

Source: Tomer and Eliason 1996: 346

aspirations for the future; a life regarded as unfulfilled may suggest that death is to be welcomed; death regarded as annihilation may bring more terror than relief. The meaning of death for a person is another complex and temporal concept which in this model is related to beliefs about the world and self. These aspects of a world-view may accord to death a fearful or blissful purpose. The significance of death to a person who believes in a cycle of rebirth, where 'life everlasting' may not be a heavenly state, will be different from what it is to someone who believes in a single span of life that leads to an eternal destiny – a common view in Britain (Davies 1996).

The religious accounts of death may be assimilated into a personal world-view and provide a means of coping with and understanding death. This explanation has provided researchers with questions about the effect of religiosity (when taken as an independent variable) on reducing death anxiety and whether facing death may enhance religiosity. The assumption that religion simply provides a consolation for death has been challenged by Bowker (1991) who argues that the origins of religion and much of the religious explorations of death have little to do with compensation. The nature and significance of death in many religions concern its value as a necessary condition of life that cannot be evaded or denied. However, much of the research in this field follows the tradition of Marx and Freud in the premise that the fear of death is the motivation for religious belief. The results of many studies, summarized by Beit-Hallahmi and Argyle (1997: 234), suggest that 'religious concern' and belief in an afterlife increase in people from the age of 60, and that older people who are religious and believe in an afterlife are better adjusted, happier and less apprehensive about death. Religious beliefs and practices concerning death require an 'investment' by people and this can be interpreted as an attempt to relieve anxiety.

Despite the abundance of thanatological research there is still much ambiguity about the way people understand and value death. The data collection instruments used in death anxiety studies tend to focus upon standardized attitudes to death (for example acceptance and anxiety) and foci of death anxiety (such as dying and afterlife), many of which are not functionally equivalent, are diverse in their theoretical grounding and have psychometric weaknesses (Neimeyer 1997). It is usually the healthy living who are asked about their anxiety and fear of death, but valid, reliable and ethical research among palliative care patients may provide useful insights into how they face death and what factors, both personal and external, may be involved. As Neimeyer concludes:

A close reading of the burgeoning literature on death anxiety points to a field of study that is more prolific than it is profound. Yet the obscurity of many of the results to date stems less from the difficulties intrinsic to studying attitudes toward death than from the methodological shortcomings that have characterized the bulk of this research. As a result of overreliance on common 'default options' – a face valid but psychometrically problematic death anxiety scale administered to a small convenience sample and correlated with a second variable having limited theoretical or practical significance – the typical study of death anxiety makes at best a modest contribution to a more adequate psychological understanding of the human encounter with death.

(Neimeyer 1997: 115)

To what extent palliative care professionals encounter patients' understanding of death and whether this goes beyond symptoms is uncertain. Few professionals (with the exception of psychological pathology) spend time in their training examining approaches to death and their own feelings and responses. Existential and spiritual issues related to death and dying may rarely surface in time-limited dialogues often aimed at assessments. A patient's attitude to death and that of carers are often presumed in institutional care, which may render the subject unnecessary and avoided. The result may be that such concerns are withheld or learnt to be irrelevant or unacceptable by patients and carers. Facing death takes people to profoundly intimate places which contain fears for most people and may ring alarm bells of vulnerability for professionals. However, being present when patients express their intimate thoughts and feelings provides the opportunity for affirmation and acceptance, challenges the isolation of suffering and creates space for meaning and growth (Barnard 1995). A personal meaning of death is not captured in discrete objective beliefs and values but will include cognitive, somatic, emotional and spiritual aspects. This is not an argument for engineering intimate encounters with patients, but a reminder that, 'Personal meaning is a fundamental dimension of personhood, and there can be no understanding of human illness or suffering without taking it into account' (Cassel 1982: 641).

Death both challenges and reinforces meaning, and people facing death may be challenged to revise the way they understand 'their' world, the way it operates and their place in it. The classic question of 'Why is this happening to me?' may be not only a cry of anguish but an indication that a person's world-view has been contradicted. Beliefs structure a person's world-view and provide familiar and dependable realities upon which life can be ventured. Anticipated and actual loss can threaten the meanings of life and the beliefs by which we interpret it. But beliefs may also enable a person to make sense of loss and find meaning in it. A small study of bereaved people who defined themselves as Christian explicitly related the meaning of their partner's death with their faith and beliefs. It was observed that this provided a predefined understanding of loss, although it did not account for all aspects of it, and there was evidence that discontinuities had prompted some reassessment of what death meant. In addition to feeling supported by their faith, the participants acknowledged uncertainties and doubts but these were understood as being contained within a spiritual framework. It appeared that religious meaning did not lessen feelings of grief and that, for some participants, whilst basic beliefs remained unquestioned, the meaning of death and the purpose of life were uncertain (Golsworthy and Coyle 1999).

The need to make, reform and reassert meaning in the face of death is the human impulse to maintain continuity when life is bereft. Health psychology and oncopsychology have models which encompass meanings and beliefs, few go as far as explicitly incorporating spiritual issues or beliefs. Palliative care is in some state of confusion over this: should it be left to a 'specialist' or is it something that anyone can and should deal with? It is difficult to establish whether or not palliative care services intentionally subordinate spirituality in seeking to help people to face death, but it is equally difficult to understand why something which can have such significant impact upon the way that death is understood is often left to chance.

The rituals of death

Palliative care cannot avoid being involved in rituals: in a general sense, rituals pervade the practice of healthcare professionals, and in an explicit sense they are necessary around the boundaries of life. As anthropology reminds us, no society is devoid of ritual, it is without equivalents and, as a basic social act, is 'requisite to the perpetuation of human social life' (Rappaport 1999: 31).

Rituals allow people to deal with ambiguities of change and give them meaning. Rituals also have an archaic association which tends to render them obscure and therefore of limited utility. The corollary is that rituals have declined because they are no longer very compatible with contemporary life. Muir challenges this thesis from an historical perspective, arguing that although the status of ritual in society has been demoted, rituals have not been abandoned but their nature has been changed.

> The modern intolerance toward 'mere ritual' originated in the ritual revolution of the sixteenth century and the deritualizations of the eighteenth. Modern rationalists have often imagined themselves to be above the delusions and obscurantism of religious rituals, even as they are oblivious to the secular rituals in which they participate. The rituals of modern mass culture have created a shifting transient sense of the sacred, now invested in political ideology, jingoistic nationalism, idealized domesticity, or endless cults, fads and ephemera. If societies demand rituals, then changing societies will produce changing rituals.
>
> (Muir 1997: 274)

Rituals of death are ubiquitous, indispensable and possibly one of the most conservative types of ritual. The functional purpose of disposal which they incorporate does not exhaust the use of ritual which interprets death by placing it within a frame of reference. This is a frame of beliefs, behaviour, meaning and conventions which allow the bereaved to deal with the calamity of loss in a contained and purposeful way. Rituals enact meaning, express beliefs, evoke emotions, represent ideals; in others words they make the invisible tangible through actions and words. Postmortem rituals therefore dramatize and emphasize death, they honour the dead and prepare and commit them to their destiny, they sanction the profoundly intense and ambivalent expressions of grief, and they place the bereaved and the dead within a social and universal context. By enabling and elaborating grief, postmortem rituals express something of the significance of the relationships which have ended and also of the sense of loss which is inherent in the mortal condition, a loss which exists because of the meaning we make of our own life and the lives of others (Marris 1986: ch. 5).

The trivial and inconsequential may be dealt with by routine, convention and repetitive actions, but rituals are used when matters of significance and profound change need to be handled. Therefore, rituals are usually distinguished from other social acts by a number of features, among them: their gravity (solemnity and formality), by the way people are involved in them (participation), by the special places and time at which they occur (context), by their use of an established order (invariance), by the means and content of their communication (formalized utterances and enduring messages), and by their powerful and convincing affect (efficacy) (Rappaport 1999: ch. 3). Rituals accomplish and achieve their purpose not directly through the physical but through the incorporeal by using meaningful words and acts which declare the significance of the ritual and convey deep connotative resonances. Rituals, unlike some other social acts, are not vague, but make explicit and clearly define what is the intention of the performance. Finally, ritual as a social act involves individuals in a collective event, establishing, guarding and bridging the boundaries between the public and private (Rappaport 1999: ch. 4).

The way in which ritual forms are employed in the history of patients and their carers range from the consultation at which the patients and carers receive the terminal diagnosis, the patients' admission for in-patient care, the declaration of death, the last offices, the funeral and memorial service. All of these significant episodes of transition are usually accompanied by the performance of established and formal orders which take place in special settings involving participation which transform that which they are imposed upon. Even if many of the examples offered here fall short of a strict definition of ritual, there are strong resemblances to ritual in that they are acts which articulate, emote, inform and redefine by enacting and communicating meaning. The point here is that palliative care makes use of 'ritual' in order to invest or impose meaning upon that which challenges and dislocates meaning, and in so doing maintains some order in the face of chaos.

At the time of death we find a number of ritual forms converging, not necessarily in any consistent pattern, to facilitate and declare the transition from life to death of the patient, to allow carers and staff to make an acknowledgement of the loss, and to convey at the very least the meaning of life now ended. But rituals of death are increasingly truncated and condensed, a result in part of the professionalization and process of death, which means that they have to carry in concentrated periods that which was once spread out over weeks. The hospice adage of 'live until you die' and the depreciated 'terminal' phase of a life-threatening illness limits the opportunities for the ritual expressions of dying for all concerned. What rituals are allowed and provided, therefore, have to work much harder and cover an area that may have been dealt with in other ways. A contemporary cremation service, in all its brevity, often feels as if it has to pick up from the moment of death, consign the body to its final resting place and take people through mourning towards life adjusted to loss in the space of twenty-five minutes.

What informs the rituals of palliative care is a mixture, as we have noted already, of traditional and detraditionalized religious beliefs, added to which are the beliefs and the 'performances' of the medical tradition. Rose (1995), for example, observed as a patient that 'cancer' means both multiplying matter and condemnation, but medicine's 'iatrogenic materiality' limited its imagination and engagement with illness such that, 'To the bearer of this news, the term "cancer" means nothing: it has no meaning. It merges without remainder into the horizon within which the difficulties, the joys, the banalities, of each day elapse' (Rose 1995: 72). As for her surgeon, she complains that:

> With a man in clerical orders, one may legitimately expect him to have faced eternity. The source of his authority will be this humility in relation to his own mortality. It should seal him from violence in love, from joining the hierarchies of exterminating angels. With a consultant surgeon, alas, you cannot expect him necessarily to have faced his own finality. Surgeons are not qualified for the one thing with which they deal: life. For they do not understand, as part of their profession, 'death', in the non-medical sense, nor therefore 'life' in the meaningful sense, inclusive of death.
>
> (Rose 1995: 72–3)

Death without meaning, death as nothing, when conveyed in ritual implies either acceptance of this by those participating in it or the ritual becoming a cipher, a meaningless act. From this emerges the important spiritual issue of what eschatology is realized in palliative care: does it stop with nihilism or does it look out towards eternity? Rose, reflecting philosophically, claims that, 'To rob life, death and language of their eternity/Does not let death go free;/It constricts it to mere vacuity' (Rose 1996: 138).

Much of the ritual response to death is a creative declaration that death is more than biological cessation for it has social, symbolic, temporal and spiritual significance. The material facts cannot be excised from more intangible dimensions, and part of ritual's efficacy is its ability to meaningfully represent values, beliefs, states and qualities in ways which substantiate and validate them. The rituals of death do not restrict it to a fatal moment for they also lift it out of its mundane timeframe and can place it in a sacred frame in which all may not be lost:

> It is as though human imagination utilizes both the drive for survival and a propensity for hopeful optimism to contradict the visible facts of life. To direct view, death brings people to a decaying end yet, against this cold fact, and in the very face of death, most human societies have asserted that life continues in another world, in a spiritual dimension or amongst the ancestral powers. But not only in an afterlife is death transcended. In this life, too, rites make it possible to lift the individual above the realm of death and decay. The human being may live as one who has died and, through contact with some higher power, now possesses some of that power to ensure that ordinary life is ordinary no longer. The words of the rites are powerful in establishing all these issues.
>
> (Davies 1997: 178)

After death

When people face death they face contradictions of finality and continuity, of absence and presence, of decay and redemption, of mortality and immortality. What the nurse pronounces as death may to the carers be a thankful release from 'this life' and to the priest be a passing from this world to the next. The plain facts of death may seem to contravene the facts of experience and the breadth of interpretations evoked by death. In particular, the religious imagination has understood death in most conceivable ways. However, death is not a question to be answered by a single universal response, there is no dichotomy in death, and people can see death both as the consequence of embodiment and the point of its departure to life beyond death, however that is conceived.

Postmortem existence can be understood on many levels but all point to transcending death, whether through personal legacies (objective and subjective), the experiences, feelings or spiritual beliefs of the bereaved and some form of 'survival' beyond the fatal event. A destiny beyond life forms part of the concept of death and may well be a significant factor in people's attitudes and response to death. In essence, a postmortem destiny concerns some future prospect for the dead person which has important consequences most immediately for the dying (in terms of preparation), the dead and those who mourn them, but also for society and the way it deals with death and those who are bereaved. As the present is a point in the human narrative that contains references to the future, any prospects held to follow from death will affect life now and modify its meaning. This has two further interrelated aspects. One concerns the continuity of the person who has died and, in particular, what form of afterlife this will take. The other concerns the 'place' in the universe for those who have died, for, to put it simply, if there is some form of postmortem survival, it must be 'located' somewhere.

This is not the only possible scenario of what happens after death, although it is a highly prominent one in many cultures. Some people have abolished any future in death and do not believe in any form of life beyond it. Personal immortality is simply an impossibility and there is no place or form of existence beyond the grave, because:

> We are physical beings and we inhabit a physical universe. If we discard the myths of self and soul and spirit, and recognise that all our life and sensation, all our capacity to think and to feel, are inextricably tied up with our bodies – if, in short, we see that we do not have bodies, we are bodies – then we might begin to realise what an extraordinary place we inhabit and what a mystery, in the true sense, life is . . . Is not that enough mystery, without your wishing to invent new mysteries of heaven and of hell?
>
> (Wilson 1995: 197)

The physicality of the person has long occupied the thoughts of theologians and philosophers, and embodiment has become something of a current preoccupation with sociologists. Death marks the breakdown of the body, and while the body may rest in the grave, it also remains a significant aspect of any postmortem survival, most obvious in the beliefs concerning the resurrection of the body, an idea that can be found in the religions of Judaism, Christianity, Islam and Zoroastrianism. These images of eventual survival beyond death refer substantially to a person's bodily identity, and it is a person of gender, appearance, activity and so forth whose presence is evoked in the recollections, memorials and experiences of the bereaved. Bodily identity therefore provides not only continuity but also a reason for a location, something which an abstract and ephemeral spirit may have no need of. More basically than this, as we have been known through our bodies, so it becomes the place of significance and meaning for others, which is one reason why it warrants utmost respect even when it is dead, and why there is usually some form of ritual performed after death even in the absence of religious rites.

Death has for some remained a future fact but without any future scenario and therefore the notion of the afterlife has lost its function. The knowledge of death is accompanied by few, if any, beliefs, but Flowers (1998) suggests that this always leaves an opening for stories and fictions, a space which is, 'even for postmodern minds, still filled with belief, namely the belief that there is no afterlife. This – the story that there is no afterlife – is the one mono-myth left in our culture, when all else is open to revision. This is the bald scenario, a story of nothing' (Flowers 1998: 55). There can be no future in nihilism and no meaning therefore derived from it: death is itself meaningless, it has no consequence, it is empty of implication and representation. Death in this bleak existential version is without a vista and the bereaved are left assuming literally nothing.

It seems reasonable to suggest that this somewhat harsh position is rarely encountered, and that for many people a belief in a form of afterlife is more common. The evidence for this is the persistent use of rituals for the dead that are premised on some form of spiritual belief, of popular expressions of the afterlife in memorials, films and books, and empirical studies. Beliefs in an afterlife are diverse and, as with other beliefs, an individual may hold what appears an incoherent set of notions about the afterlife, acquired unsystematically, and appearing somewhat inconsistent and disorganized. Davies underlines the importance of recognizing this and emphasizes that, 'logical contradiction need not necessarily worry individuals whose varied views are drawn on for different purposes and in different contexts' (Davies 1997: 151). In facing death, a person may for the first time be prompted into formulating their beliefs about death, and have to make choices based upon them: 'Would you like us to call the chaplain to say some prayers before your aunt dies?' 'Do we need to observe any particular requirements in preparing her body?' 'Whom would you like to conduct the funeral service?' These may be questions not only for the deceased but also for the dying who wish to prepare for their death, and may have particularly important consequence for those of certain faiths and traditions. Those who support the dying and bereaved may not have thought through their beliefs either, and a proper reticence that wards against imposing beliefs may frustrate what could be a helpful or necessary exploration of the afterlife.

It is in the religious exploration of death that we discover some of the most significant, enduring and hopeful beliefs concerning what happens after death. As we might expect, what religion implies about 'human nature and its destiny is by no means trivial or ill-considered; still less is it only a product of abject wishful thinking, or of cynical exploitation of the credulous' (Bowker 1991: 211). We have already noted a general attribute that religion gives to death, that death is necessary for life, but the religious exploration also affirms that there is a continuity of a person's identity despite death's disruption. A belief in an indestructible soul, resurrection, rebirth, reincarnation or the attainment of an eternal tranquil state all suggest an ultimate destiny for humanity beyond death (Badham 1995). Differences in these beliefs are not negligible and become evident in the customs and rituals surrounding death, in the concepts used and in the pathways to an ultimate destiny (Bowker 1983: ch. 10). But what can perhaps be made as a more general point is that the religious beliefs about human destiny are remarkably pervasive, durable and adaptable. Reincarnation, for example, is not part of the Christian concept of the afterlife, but Davies has found that 12 per cent of people in Britain claim some belief in the idea of the dead 'coming back as something else' (Davies 1997: 152). Globalization, the lack of a prevailing orthodoxy and the presence of different faith communities have contributed to many people assimilating various postmortem beliefs.

The New Age movement and many of the 'new' religions often have un-developed although eclectic eschatologies concentrating upon the development and perfection of the true self which is beyond death's destruction. The utopianism of New Age philosophies suggests the transcendence of the ego and attaining a heaven on earth. Death for New Agers is not to be feared but to be mastered, because 'death is the way to life and the subtext is that as god, the individual is responsible for determining the manner and content of both' (Clarke 1995: 136). Death can also be approached from a humanist perspective which does not invoke the sacred or eternal or rely upon metaphysics. The focus of meaning is in the life that has been lived and in the example that can be continued. The ritual form concerns the celebration of the deceased person and is inevitably life-centred. The funeral therefore becomes the concluding chapter of the person's history rather than the rite of transition that the person may have made to another life.

The 'ultimate' destiny of a person with a terminal illness is not something that forms an explicit part of palliative care philosophy. The respect for individual autonomy leaves services open to accommodate almost any personal belief and practice, with in-patient services providing a neutral territory for customs, rituals and views within the limits of tolerance. But the meaning of death to a patient and their carers seems too significant for it to be left unacknowledged and for some unexplored. As with other spiritual aspects this may be another example of professionals maintaining silence because of their own unexplored beliefs and their uncertain comprehension of this dimension. What death means to the professional may be unspoken but it will not be absent in their approach to dealing with death or inoperative from the way they understand the people they care for and witness dying. When it comes to the support of the bereaved, palliative care services display much less reticence about being involved. The potential pathology that grief may represent or the precarious course that the bereaved have to navigate is clear justification to some that intervention is necessary. Seale observes that:

> It is probably true to say . . . that the medicalisation of grief, constructing it as a potential psychiatric problem for which active intervention is necessary to move people towards good adjustment, has been more intense than any parallel medicalisation of the inner experience of dying. This may be because psychiatry plays a part in the broader social institution of medicine, with concerns to regulate populations of the living and reproduce existing social relations. The dying present a less pressing political problem than those with lives yet to lead, with all the potential for disorder and trouble that the living can present. This is not to say that dying has not been constituted as involving psychological disorder, but this coexists with a number of other disease-related and spiritual problems that are less noted among the bereaved.
>
> (Seale 1998: 194)

The aim of grief work (still substantially Freudian) is to achieve disengagement and detachment from the dead, resolution of the conflicting emotions surrounding loss and a return to life having adapted and adjusted to this severe change (Walter 1999). The spiritual aspect of grief will probably involve the beliefs of the bereaved and those known of the dead person in postmortem destiny, allowing that the two may not necessarily be consistent. 'Is the one who has died now at peace?' 'Able to see me?' 'Reunited with other members of the family who have died?' 'Reborn as what?' The answers to these types of question will have a bearing on mourning and, with the probable exception of nihilists, may assist in the relocation of the deceased (Worden 1991) rather than their abandonment. The Harvard Child Bereavement Study has found that maintaining an ongoing relationship with a dead parent is a normal part of the 'constructing' process in which the parent is internally represented, the meaning of loss is reinterpreted in an ongoing way and the deceased is memorialized (Worden 1996). The study reported that:

> Constructing a connection to the deceased is a process that involves family members talking about the loss. Highly connected children tended to come from families that were rated closer and more cohesive. These families experienced lower levels of stress and there was an emphasis on religious and spiritual support. In such families both the surviving parent and the child were willing to talk about, to memorialize, and to relocate the lost member as part of the family process.
>
> (Worden 1996: 32)

Many religious traditions not only have locations for the deceased but also ritually remember the dead and their place in the community of the living. Perhaps counselling and support for the bereaved can provide, for those without such beliefs or access to such resources, a 'community' in which to explore the meaning of death, the experience of grief and an opportunity to address the social isolation that can accompany mourning. In addition, the bereaved may memorialize the dead through sharing of stories and group activities. For in whatever way the dead do not disappear, their presence is felt, and it is this insistence in mourning that saves us from dishonouring the dead and uprooting the meanings that life has invested in them.

A common thread has been running through this chapter: the need of humanity to maintain meaning in life. Death, as the most profound challenge to meaning, has forced humanity endlessly to ponder this life in the knowledge of finitude and to deal meaningfully with death. Palliative care is one such response to death, arising from a desire to reform a benighted terminal care and to address dying as more than a biomedical process. What is critical to this enterprise has to be what is understood by being human, its mortality and its destiny, without which death remains a physical event dissociated from any further meaning. Thankfully, only in its most depraved times has humankind treated death as nothing more than this. Whether through religion, philosophy or the arts, people have insisted that death matters and that it has significance beyond the inevitable ending it imposes. This is the horizon that anyone involved in the care of the dying, the handling of the dead and the support of the bereaved looks out upon – an endless vista of beliefs and meanings constructed by those subject to death. As with ritual, it is a human expression that palliative care cannot avoid or disregard.

4 | Who cares for the spirit?

Palliative care makes a claim to comprehensibility both in terms of its whole-person approach and in its relevance to all care settings along the patient's pathway. Spiritual care is most explicitly described as part of palliative care provision provided in specialist services (NCHSPCS 1995) but there are also expectations from other services, such as cancer services, that spiritual care will be available (Calman and Hine 1995: 20). Historically, spiritual care of the dying was the domain of religious communities most notably in their hospices along the pilgrim routes to the Holy Land. The Knights Hospitallers of the Order of St John of Jerusalem, the Benedictines and the Irish Sisters of Charity are other examples of the religious foundations of care provided for the sick, needy and dying. This legacy has influenced the distinctive philosophy of palliative care and firmly rooted the spiritual within the encompassing provision of care. This spiritual aspect provides palliative care with one of its distinctive and possibly more problematic characteristics. Stoddard (1979) claims that it is this difference which underpins not only the rationale for palliative care but the inspiration for those who work in this field:

> The hospice movement . . . is firmly rooted in reality. The facts of human life are its base: physical facts, psychological facts, historical facts, economic facts, and not least of all, the fact that spiritual forces are at work in us constantly, however little we may be aware of them. The hospice process, whatever its location, its staffing and funding problems, or the stage of development reached by a particular facility, is faith in action. Humanists may prefer to call it faith in humanity; atheists may insist that it has nothing to do with God; and many people within the movement itself are willing to work for the comfort

of the dying without believing in any sort of afterlife. Nevertheless, faith is the heart of this process and this profession, simply because there is no other force (by whatever name) that could cause people to behave toward one another as they do in the hospice situation. Physical care of those who are 'failing' can be bought and paid for. 'Useless' members of society can be dealt with by legislation, revolution, or simple elimination. The energy for hospice work, however, must come from an entirely different source.

(Stoddard 1979: 195)

If the church provided terminal care in the past with its concomitant care of the soul, it is the National Health Service and voluntary sector which provide nearly all palliative care today which is generally careful to avoid any explicit references to religion with the exception of saintly iconography and dedications. It is uncertain how many services would regard themselves as 'faith in action' in the way that Stoddard interprets it; and without questioning the commitment of the staff who work in this field, most people have plausibly mixed motives for the choices they make. However, what is often referred to as the 'special quality' of palliative care is in no small way associated with a possibly romantic if not useful expectation that staff are exceptional. If they were not why should people entrust themselves or those significant to them to their hands? Equally, if dying and death have a spiritual quality and aspect, it is surely important to assume that those who deal with terminal illness are sensitive to this and capable of responding to it. As the roots of faith are trust and belief, it does not seem unreasonable, therefore, for the dying to have trust in those who care for them and for palliative care professionals to believe that what they do matters.

Premodern hospice care was set firmly within a religious context where the ministries of the church were an integral feature of a community of explicit faith. Today the context is avowedly secular, with a general responsibility for spiritual care resting with the multidisciplinary team but often with specific duties allocated to some form of chaplaincy. The contemporary community is a heterogeneous composition of many faiths, a breadth of spiritual orientations and a wide range of beliefs. When this is combined with an indefinite concept of spiritual care there can be an inevitable confusion as to who provides spiritual care and how the responsibility is discharged, which is only compounded by feelings of apprehension and uncertainty. Care, however, is in essence a practical and interpersonal endeavour: it requires organizing; responsibilities and accountability need to be identified and resources allocated. But more fundamental than this is the issue of whether spirituality can be distinguished sufficiently to warrant uniqueness and whether it constitutes part of the patient's good which palliative care aims to promote in its totality.

Recognizing a need

Clinical pathology is the cornerstone of much health care which is organized substantially around diagnostic techniques and their consequences. This is a process of determining what action should be taken according to indicators of disease and a metric of illness. Interventions are designed to restore a person to health, to correct a malfunction or to repair what is broken. As an approach it relies largely upon a restricted hermeneutic which sees a person as a natural object and biological organism accessible to examination and investigation. By measuring what it can, biomedicine aims to find an empirical cause of illness and thereby redress its damaging effects with physical and pharmaceutical treatments. In this paradigm, therefore, a need is defined by a loss of function and the presence of objective disease, and a need is addressed by the practical application of theoretical knowledge in the form of standardized interventions. This highly successful approach has become the dominant model of much health care, and whilst it provides a precedent for palliative care it is generally regarded as a part of the care offered and a particular contribution to the overall quality of patients' lives. This is why the needs of patients in palliative care are conceived with such breadth, but there are other, more fundamental distinctions which have a bearing on the provision of spiritual care.

Need in a general sense means a lack of something or a want, and it may be of sufficient moral weight to oblige others to respond to it in a dutiful way. Needs arise in two distinct ways: firstly, there are generic needs that exist because we are human; secondly, there are needs which arise because of our individual aims. Basic needs, as opposed to instrumental needs, are taken to be a requisite of living and not a matter of individual choice, that is why they are frequently associated with the strong moral claim of obligation. Health care is provided in part on this basis because in order simply to live we have a basic need for health. But while this concept of need is generally accepted, it remains indeterminate, for what type or level of health do we need and who is to say what contributes simply to living. Culturally specific convention usually dictates the standards of basic human need, the minimum levels of nutrition, liberty, education and so forth that are considered necessary for the existence of a human being. But this rests upon the notion of what is of value and to whom, which is why desires, by contrast, are usually afforded a much weaker purchase on the response by others because they are often the result of individual choice and they do not necessarily coincide with those of society (Griffin 1986: ch. 3).

In palliative care the basic need of health is often elusive and certainly limited. Indeed, health in the usual sense may not matter as much as other values to a person close to death. The difference can be described as a distinction between objective and subjective standards, where the objective is regarded as generic and the subjective is contingent upon an individual's circumstances, plans, commitments and interests, although we have to allow that subjective standards may be widely imitated. In palliative care, subjective standards are considered to have great weight, hence the focus of palliative care is the individual patient and how that person can be enabled to live and die with a terminal disease in such a way that respects the individual's interests. An objective standard may be to treat pain but a person may decide to forgo additional morphine in order to be sure to take part in a marriage service. Chemotherapy may hold out the possibility of prolonging life, but a person may prefer a honeymoon without nausea and hair loss.

It is evident that the interests of a person are usually afforded greater consideration when that person is known to be dying than when they are expected to recover from their illness. One reason for this comes from the preciousness associated with the remaining days of life such that the opportunities for satisfying the dying person's interests are likely to be decreasing. By contrast, and within limits, any lack of consideration or any disregard by carers for the interests of a person whose injured condition is only temporary is unlikely to have a serious impact upon the overall aims of that person's life. Clearly this is not the case for dying patients who may become increasingly dependent upon others for their interests to be regarded and acted upon. This suggests a greater awareness and sensitivity to the broad concerns and interests of patients in palliative care.

Spirituality rarely appears in the accounts of general health care for it is regarded as too subjective, is not afforded much moral weight and is a personal interest considered to have little consequence in an episode of care. In palliative care, however, spirituality is accepted not only as a legitimate aspect of being human – an ontological good – but also as one which may provide meaning and value to a person whose very life is being challenged. However, what is the lack or need that must be addressed? Certainly we can argue that the expression of a person's spirituality may require facilities and personnel, but more than this is the argument that nurturing and supporting a person's spirituality will contribute to their fundamental interest or good.

Not all patients' interests can be considered harmless or beneficial, which is why promoting the patient's *best* interests is a necessary condition. Some interests are plainly more valuable to a person than others, and Dworkin has usefully described these as critical interests which embrace those preferential values to which a person is most committed, aspires, and which can lead to self-defining decisions (Dworkin 1993: 201–5). Critical interests concern people because they are in some way basic or vital to who they are, and are expressed through the needs and preferences that constitute a person's convictions. A patient may therefore decline drugs which reduce pain but as a consequence increases drowsiness in order to pray. Another patient may express a clear wish to die because of their conviction in an afterlife free from pain. The values, meanings and beliefs of people govern and direct their critical interests and their decisions and therefore express something of their spiritual orientation. Consequently the need for spiritual care is not only about what is required to facilitate spiritual practices but also about promoting the patient's good through actively practising the art of attending to the patient's world-view including life's meaning and ultimate destiny. This attention is not an ancillary task but one that is central to establishing the value of the person and the interests which the patient holds in trust with carers.

Compared with disease pathology, the argument of need presented so far lacks comparable precision, although spiritual care is not unique in this. Clinical medicine and other disciplines do not rely upon diagnostic tests to identify need. Using Bradshaw's (1972) taxonomy we can describe four interrelated approaches to need. 'Normative need' is determined by the professional and is indicated by an unacceptable differential between the actual and the desirable. What is desirable is based upon standards formulated by experts and provides a benchmark against which to measure the individual. This is the form of needs assessment employed in a wide range of care practices and some attempt at this has been made in spiritual care. 'Felt need' is determined by individuals being assessed to receive a service. These subjective views are contingent upon personal perceptions, knowledge, and the trust and confidence to disclose them. There is a limited amount of research available concerning patients' views on spiritual care. When felt need is translated into a demand it becomes an 'expressed need'. Not all felt needs become expressed as demand as they may be subject to disincentives and there may be no actual or possible service available to meet the need. The reverse of this is that the presence of a service may generate demand. Finally, 'comparative need' is determined by differentials of service between comparable individuals or groups. A new palliative care unit may therefore cite the services of a similar unit to justify an equivalent provision. This is an argument frequently used for the provision of chaplaincy alongside other disciplines. The need for spiritual care may not be demonstrable in the way that the need for a blood transfusion is from a simple blood test. But then so much of the care that is offered to people lies outside objective measures and aims to address needs that are difficult to register in ways that can be interpreted reliably away from the patient's narrative.

Need is both experienced and observed, and results from social, psychological and spiritual as well as biological sequelae. The concern in palliative care for all the dimensions of personhood and its commitment to patient well-being and quality of life means that it has to go beyond the limits of medicine's technical skills. Symptoms may present themselves in a way that can be measured, but well-being does not manifest itself in this way, it is elusive:

It is not something which invites or demands permanent attention. Rather it belongs to that miraculous capacity we have to forget ourselves. But then what does theory, this pure 'looking on', seek to discover? What does it find? Here we speak of the problem of the body and the soul. We are confident that we know what the body is, but nobody knows what the soul is. What is the relationship between the body and the soul? Some kind of dynamic interrelationship perhaps? We can say that the body is life, that which is alive, and that the soul is what enlivens or animates. Yet both are so profoundly interrelated that every attempt to objectify either of them without the other in the end leads to absurdity.

(Gadamer 1996: 96)

The enthusiastic and uncritical use of assessment tools and instruments to measure need must not make us indifferent to those unrationalized elements of being human and the wider considerations of care which are recognized not so much by diligence or genius as by compassion and wisdom. The spiritual domain is to a large extent plainly undemonstrable, but this does not remove it from the view of palliative care, careful research, professional competence, the practicalities of providing a service or our encounters with others. The need for spiritual care has an impressive historical legacy, it is a recurrent theme in the contemporary explorations of many disciplines and it remains a domain which can take us closer to what it means to be human even in the face of death.

Chaplains

However convincing the preceding arguments are for recognizing spiritual need, there can be few palliative care services that do not include chaplaincy within their multidisciplinary teams specifically to meet this need. The National Health Service has since its inception included provision for the spiritual needs of patients and staff in the form of chaplains, and most of the charitable services have followed this practice. Chaplains are predominantly Anglican priests, which reflects to some extent the identification of the majority of patients with the Church of England and its representative role in the religious life of the nation. But chaplains have a broader remit to all patients acquired through the institutional role. This allows chaplains to cross community boundaries and church conventions to exercise a responsibility to people of any or no faith, although particular patients' needs may be met through chaplains from denominations and faith communities corresponding to those of the patient.

The role of the chaplain provides us with some insight into the institutional response to spiritual needs, for it is the chaplain who has the specific professional duty of the spiritual care of patients, carers and staff. How this duty is discharged will depend upon a wide range of factors, for the role has no generic description, it exists only 'locally' in the relationship be-tween the person appointed and the expectations and demands of a service. A major defining factor is the approach that the chaplain takes to illness, dying and death, something which can vary. This derives from such things as training, the theological perspective held, the individual's experience and professional formation, skills and personality. Another significant factor is how the chaplain relates to the other members of the interdisciplinary team, which can be particularly important given the part-time nature of many chaplaincy posts. This is a matter of group dynamics and culture as much as of the structure and operation of the team. This organizational context influences how much the chaplain is integrated into the team, the assump-tions made about the role and what use is made of the chaplain. These factors are not unique to the chaplain's role but they are probably more prominent given the lone position of the role.

Chaplains, as with other professionals, are usually expected to be self-directed in their work although available for referrals. The relatively small number of people in an in-patient service means that a chaplain can be familiar with all patients from which a caseload can be discerned. Day units and community services limit this possibility and a chaplain may need to rely upon colleagues for referrals. This is complemented by requests from patients and their carers to see the chaplain. Without direct contact with patients chaplains must rely upon other disciplines to be their agents and to broker referrals. This intermediary will need to have a grasp of the chaplain's role and of the potential benefit to a patient as well as suitable assessment and communication skills to make an effective referral.

Beckford and Gilliat (1996), in their research into healthcare chaplains, outlined several main categories into which chaplains ranked their major tasks:

> Being available to listen, visit wards and assess patients' spiritual needs had the highest priority. Conducting worship, taking services and doing advocacy on behalf of individual patients came next in the order of importance. Liaising with staff, other clergy and health care managers was ranked slightly ahead of providing support for families and other carers.
>
> (Beckford and Gilliat 1996: 24)

In palliative care, both teamwork and the greater inclusion of carers are likely to vary this pattern such that family support and liaising with staff would attain a higher priority. In addition, chaplains may be involved with the wider activities of a palliative care service, including bereavement support, education, policy development and staff support. These tasks can expand the scope of the role and enable the chaplain to be involved with many aspects of the service and at a number of different levels. This involvement can reinforce a comprehensive approach to spirituality and ensure that spirituality is represented in forums which can influence its credibility and validation. In parallel to this, such involvement can help to establish the value of the chaplain's role among peers.

The chaplain's role is substantially patient-focused and its primary purpose is the provision of spiritual care. This can be described in essence as a process of interaction founded upon an empathic relationship in which the spiritual dimension is acknowledged and opportunity is given for spiritual issues to be explored. The process is to some extent psychological, and in this sense it is similar to counselling, but it is not exclusively so, because the frame of reference is that of the spiritual. This difference is further emphasized by the understanding brought to spiritual care of what it means to be human. This includes issues of belief, value, meaning and transcendence which may also open the frame to metaphysical or supernatural aspects. In addition, as a member of a faith community, the chaplain 'enjoys freedom, but not compulsion, to draw upon the traditional resources of the community of faith such as prayers, scripture and sacrament, the needs, stated or perceived, of the person receiving care being determinative' (Lyall 1998: 18). This process may be considered therapeutic in that it may enable a person to address existential concerns, support the search for meaning and help the person to face mortality. A seminal expression of this approach was given by Autton (1975) before pallaitive care became established:

> It is not for the chaplain to discuss the medical chances of survival, which is the task of the doctor. It is, however, his function to *relate*, to *accept*, and to *listen*. In this way he will be able to diagnose some of the basic fears uppermost in the patient's mind. He will pay far more attention to feelings rather than words, watching with gentleness and listening with attention and respect. He can be asking himself such questions about some of the spiritual and emotional needs of the patient. 'Who is this person to whom I am ministering?' 'How is he responding to his present predicament?' 'What are some of his special spiritual needs at this time?' The chaplain, in recognising some of the feelings and demands of the sufferer, can then help him to *absorb*, *interpret*, and *transcend* them, so that the temporal eventually becomes transformed into the eternal.
>
> (Autton 1975: 108)

It may be thought that the chaplain must operate on another 'plane' when dealing with spiritual needs, but this ignores the plain fact that most people do not express their spirituality through the ephemeral or mystical but in the concrete and mundane realities of their history, relationships, plans and decisions as well as in their hopes and fears. This is where the task of hermeneutics becomes evident and is one which is shared between patient and chaplain. Speck (1998) suggests that a coherent approach to this can be gained from the perspectives of the past, present and future which can allow patients to review their life, explore what being ill means to them and express their longings for their remaining life and their concerns about dying and death (Speck 1998: 805–14).

Patients who have a religious orientation, however dormant, may find in the chaplain a convenient resource in facilitating their faith practices. If the patient and chaplain are from the same faith community there is the possibility of the chaplain meeting religious needs, or, if not, making a referral with the patient's consent to an appropriate colleague or member of the respective faith community. This scope of coordinating the provision of religious care for people of different faiths will be indicated to some extent by the communities which come within the boundaries of the palliative care service. The involvement of ministers from different faith communities is usually no more than an informal arrangement, and this raises the questions of their accessibility and the equity of the service provided. There are also broader issues concerning the ethnic and cultural diversity of patients and their carers and the implications this has for aspects of a service such as patients' dietary requirements or the observance of festivals. This diversity means that the chaplain has a responsibility for ensuring that matters of faith are addressed within the organization and that, when it is required, there is the mechanism for making referrals to representatives of different faith communities. The corollary is that some palliative care services may serve communities for whom a Christian chaplain is clearly inappropriate.

Spiritual care is patient-focused but it will extend to those who are significant to patients who may want to explore their past, present and future in the light of their relationship to the patient. This can bring opportunities to discern and express the value and meaning of the relationship (positive and negative), explore issues of belief and contemplate a future in the anticipation and actuality of the death of a person who is a part of their life. Some of this may be presented in practical issues such as how to mark a significant anniversary, what to tell children, or asking for advice on arranging a funeral or memorial service. The chaplain may become a religious resource for a carer who has become dislocated from a faith community, or may facilitate links with local resources. A chaplain may also be the member of the multidisciplinary team who is asked to facilitate arbitration in social conflicts, provide advocacy for the patient or represent disregarded interests. This is where the association of chaplain with 'social worker' becomes apparent and attests to the independent position that some regard the chaplain to occupy in terms of both a patient's relationships and the provision of physical care.

The spiritual care provided by a chaplain will include the ritual form, at the very least in terms of religious rites practised. As we have discussed, rituals through words and actions make the invisible visible. In representing and validating the intangible, a ritual form may assist a patient or those significant to them to express values, meanings and beliefs. Conducting a service of holy communion, the blessing of a relationship, the saying of commendatory prayers at the time of death and conducting a patient's funeral may all be occasions where the chaplain performs ritual, whatever the extent of the religious content. There is also the chaplain's contribution to the extrinsic public rituals of the organization, such as the memorial services which palliative care units frequently provide for the bereaved, and the organization's intrinsic professional 'rituals' such as ward rounds, case conferences and debriefings following the death of a patient.

It is inevitable, as well as a professional duty, that chaplains include staff within their compass of spiritual care, as staff too are faced with spiritual issues. It is a contention of this book that many healthcare professionals generally have few opportunities to develop an appreciation of the spiritual dimension of a human being beyond their own experiences and spiritual orientation. Equally, there are probably few explicit opportunities among staff to explore the impact on their own spirituality of caring for people with life-threatening illnesses and to reflect upon the spiritual dimension of the care they provide. A chaplain may be a catalyst and facilitator for such discussions through contributing to case meetings, debriefing of care teams, training programmes and individual consultations.

Nurses

The professionals who have the greatest patient contact in most services are nurses, and the nursing profession is increasingly exploring all dimensions of care, including the spiritual. Grey (1994) represents the views put forward in much nursing literature in this field when she advocates that, 'if palliative care nurses are to practise true holistic care, then it is vital to consider the spiritual aspects by enabling and supporting each person to acknowledge their spirituality, revise it as necessary, and affirm it in daily living and dying' (Grey 1994: 216). Spirituality, it is argued, is an aspect of the patient and therefore comes within the boundary of nursing care. It can therefore be subject to nursing models, assessed and taken as 'a basis for therapeutic intervention either by providing counselling personally . . . or by referral to others such as chaplains, the religious visiting services or other counsellors' (Bown and Williams 1993: 61).

Encompassing the whole of a person in care is something of a nursing ideal in which spirituality can be included as a constituent part. Oldnall (1996), in a critical review of 26 theories, reported that whilst 14 briefly acknowledged the spiritual domain in their frameworks, only Watson's contained adequate explanation and only Watson's and Neuman's 'acknowledged the impact of spirituality in the development of their respective theories' (Oldnall 1996: 140). More typical is the popular model of Roper, Logan and Tierney (Roper *et al.* 1996) which draws upon Maslow's theory of hierarchical human needs. The goal of this theory is a fully functioning (self-actualizing) person whose instinctive tendencies are towards wholeness that can be promoted by satisfying the person's more basic needs for such things as survival, safety and belonging thus providing the context in which the person may develop. In the Roper–Logan–Tierney model, religious worship is recognized as an activity of daily living, but this is often translated into the practical task of enquiring after a patient's religious affiliation upon admission.

The nursing process concerns the planning and delivery of care which depends upon assessing needs, making appropriate interventions and evaluating the outcome. This requires a conceptual knowledge of spirituality, hermeneutic skills and an ability to utilize effective responses. In a study of 685 nurses, Ross (1994) reported that the nurses defined spiritual needs in a way that was consistent with the literature but that they had a tendency to understand it in religious terms. The majority of nurses indicated that they had identified spiritual needs using a variety of indicators, 70 per cent of which were recognized through non-verbal means of communication and observation. Nearly all the nurses considered themselves to be responsible for responding to the spiritual needs of patients, but for more than half of them this meant referring to others. Interventions were evaluated mainly through reassessing the original non-verbal cues (Ross 1994: 442–5).

Accurate assessment of needs is pivotal to the nursing process, but it is significant that generally nurses in Ross's study did not involve patients directly in either the assessment of spiritual need or the effectiveness of interventions aimed at these needs. This raises the important question of the validity of this interpretation of these spiritual needs when this interpretation is derived solely from patients' signs. The ideal clearly envisages that a thorough assessment relies upon understanding the spiritual experiences and expressions of a patient. For this to be achieved, nurses must move beyond observation and enter into dialogue with patients. However, Heaven and Maguire (1997) report that patients in hospices not only appear much less willing to disclose psychological, social and spiritual concerns to nurses but may deliberately withhold such information. This hospice study of 44 nurses and 87 patients affirmed the view that inadequate communication skills lead to presumptions about patients' needs; it also cited difficulties of recognizing patient concerns and documenting them. Heaven and Maguire suggest that non-disclosure may be a consequence of the hospice emphasis on symptom control through which patients 'learn' that professionals are not interested in other issues. In addition, patients may want to demonstrate that they are coping or they may not want to burden staff who appear vulnerable. But the study clearly showed that 'nondisclosure cannot be interpreted as a lack of concerns or distress – indeed those patients who were most depressed or anxious were found to be most likely to withhold their concerns' (Heaven and Maguire 1997: 283–90).

Patients may quickly ascertain whether they are going to be able to entrust their concerns to particular members of staff. This will depend not only on the use of good communication skills by staff but also the ability of staff to convey to patients that an holistic philosophy is integrated into practice and that they are not only interested but also capable of understanding and responding to the spiritual domain. A patient is unlikely to share spiritual issues with a professional who appears to be insensitive to them, as Rose (see Chapter 3) demonstrated. The beliefs and values of professionals matter in this respect, and it seems reasonable to suggest that the chaplain who obviously operates in the spiritual domain may be the appropriate person with whom to share concerns and hopes. Similarly, the chaplain plainly does not have a focus upon physical symptoms and may be regarded as interested in the non-physical aspects of the person. But these arguments may well apply to other members of the multidisciplinary team who are not implicated in the process of physical diagnosis and intervention, or who obviously do not represent an expression of faith that may present a barrier to a patient.

Grey (1994) asserts that there is 'little practical guidance available for nurses who wish to understand a patient's spiritual needs and resources. However, if an holistic approach is to be practised, ignoring the spiritual aspects of patients' lives is an omission of care' (Grey 1994: 219). The ideal is by admission rarely approached but the responsibility is affirmed. This discrepancy is explained by a number of significant factors which may include:

- a narrow conceptualization and poor awareness of spirituality
- fear of incompetence
- uncertainty regarding personal spiritual and religious beliefs and values
- discomfort with the conditions that frequently bring spiritual needs to the surface
- disagreement that spirituality is within the domain of nursing care
- the nursing process
- lack of time, low priority
- deficiencies in communication skills
- a focus on physical needs
- low nurse/patient ratio
- environmental factors
- patient's mental state and physical condition
- failure to integrate spiritual care issues into the nursing process

(based upon Taylor *et al.* 1995: 31)

Spirituality represents a recognized challenge for nursing care; it also exemplifies an issue in the development of nursing as a profession, for an ambiguous concept with limited systematic theory may hinder the aim of nursing to attain a professional status equal to that of the medical disciplines. It has been a contentious issue in that it has highlighted the shift in nursing away from its religious foundation. Bradshaw (1996a) charts a sea-change in nursing philosophy during the 1970s which she interprets as the revision of nursing tradition in favour of liberal humanism at the expense of its historical theological and pastoral base. The emerging sociocultural and existential approaches to nursing are presented by Bradshaw as undermining the spiritual ethic of nursing care without which nursing becomes a matter of technique, skills and knowledge rather than a covenant service of care. The 'Nightingale' model of faithful nursing, however, appears to retain a limited appeal to a discipline with strong professional aspirations, an expanding academic discourse and a secular world-view. But spiritual care, far from being abandoned, has been rediscovered and reinterpreted so that it becomes a further example of the knowledge and role of the nurse. This has stimulated various efforts to gain insight into spirituality which has required critical reflection upon the conceptual basis of nursing, an examination of nursing experience and the assumption that spirituality can, to a useful extent, be identified, described and applied to practice. As Reed (1992) optimistically comments:

> The discipline of nursing has not retreated from challenges of investigating complex human phenomena, and the area of spirituality is no exception. Attempts to understand spirituality, or any human phenomenon, can be limited by the conceptual machinery of the discipline. However, nursing has a rich knowledge base from conceptual, empirical, and clinical sources that can be organized to support an epistemologic foundation for the study of spirituality. Explicating this paradigm on spirituality may facilitate continued investigation and knowledge development in nursing by providing a perspective for inquiry while stimulating critical dialogue.
>
> (Reed 1992: 355)

Nursing embraces spirituality conceptually and there is a strong assumption that the nursing role in palliative care should embrace spiritual care. In practice, a number factors mitigate against nurses fulfilling this role, not least the diagnostic process which nursing emulates. When acting as patient guardians, nurses can be the critical factor in drawing upon the skills of other team members and in ensuring that the spiritual interests of patients are represented in the planning and provision of care. More fundamentally, spirituality has become an issue for nursing in its evolution because it prompts a clarification of what constitutes the art of nursing and the nature of the human condition which it believes it is caring for. It is also a domain which may enhance or embarrass this emerging profession which, at present, may explain why on this issue it stands in an ambiguous relationship to other professionals, and to chaplains in particular.

Spiritual care and the team approach

The collaborative use of complementary skills and knowledge within a team is widely recognized as providing the necessarily comprehensive perspective to achieve quality palliative care. In aiming to meet the whole needs of patients and their carers it is usual that a number of different expertise and roles will be required and this constitutes the varying composition of a patient-centred team. It has been suggested that most core teams in palliative care consist of a physician, chaplain, nurse and social worker, consulting with and involving other members of the wider team (Ajemian 1993). Whatever the make-up of the team, it is important that there is agreement on particular responsibilities and clarification of roles in order for care to be coordinated, timely and effective in addressing the patient's needs.

Spiritual care, as with other aspects of palliative care, cannot be left to caprice. Care is a practical matter, it requires organizing and responsibilities need to be identified and assigned. The administration of medication, for example, is defined as a function of particular grades of nurses within the team and the responsibility of specific individuals at any given time who are accountable for fulfilling the task. The social worker may be assigned the task of talking with the patient's partner about concerns regarding their children. The responsibility is in part a function of the recognized competence of the practitioner (the office held) and the sanction granted them by the team and the wider society to perform the task (the authority assigned). As Lucas (1993) recognizes, 'Responsibility and duty are correlative: if I am to have responsibility for something, I have to have the authority and power to act so as to discharge it' (Lucas 1993: 182). But can there be a responsibility for spiritual care and can it be defined above a general consideration in order to identify specific duties? Any ambiguity in the answers obtained to these questions is reproduced in the ambiguities of roles and the confusion of responsibilities.

A palliative care service recognizes a responsibility to provide care by meeting the needs of patients; it discharges this responsibility through specific duties. Responsibility is central to our moral thinking and fundamental to patient care for it is a demonstration of the moral probity that enables people to place their trust in a palliative care service. Responsibility also applies to inaction or omission in that a person may be held accountable for a failure to act in a certain way, especially if it is the case of an explicit duty assigned as a result of taking on a particular role. This is the argument presented by Grey (1994) when she considers the failure of nurses to account for the spiritual dimension. It is premised on the claim that spiritual care constitutes part of the nurse's duty. However, a duty that is vague cannot be clarified any further in a responsibility, and so the case becomes weaker in its moral purchase. Equally it is difficult to see that the responsibility for spiritual care can reside more generally with the team unless it is incorporated into some form of general duty of care – an issue we discuss in the next chapter. Palliative care's specification of the spiritual dimension and its care provision render it a more exact obligation, although, as with many interpersonal tasks, there is a limit to the level of precision by which it can be defined. However, actions directed at fulfilling this obligation must bear greater moral evaluation and accountability because of its distinction. As an example of what spiritual care implies, let us consider the outline framework given by Twycross and Lack (1990) which is intended primarily to direct a doctor:

> It is important to discover what the patient's spiritual needs are. Whether apparent or not, most patients are in need of spiritual help and are seeking answers to questions such as:
>
> - *The meaning of life*: What is the meaning of life in a time of serious illness?
> - *Value systems*: What value is there in money, material possessions, and social position?
> - *Meaning of suffering and pain*: Why do I have to suffer? Why do I have to have pain?
> - *Guilt feelings*: I have done many wrong things; how can they be corrected? How can I be forgiven?
> - *Quest after God*: Is there a God? Why does God allow me to suffer like this?
> - *Life after death*: Is there life after death? How can I believe in life after death?
>
> Only a minority of patients discuss the spiritual aspects of life and death with their doctor. The majority do so with another team member, with relative or close friends.
>
> - It is important to recognize that the dying do consider such issues and be able to respond sympathetically if a patient chooses to raise them.
> - Patients are very perceptive, they are unlikely to embarrass a doctor if they sense that communication at this level will cause discomfort.
> - A doctor's prime responsibility is to help maintain an environment which is supportive of the patient. This requires control of symptoms so that the patient is able to consider these issues.
> - When appropriate, the doctor should alert the chaplain, priest, or rabbi to the fact that: 'Mr X is seriously ill and may appreciate a visit'.
>
> Regard for the patient as an individual does not allow the imposition of one's faith, or lack of it, on him. Many patients are comforted by the discovery that their doctor has a religious faith.
>
> (Twycross and Lack 1990: 208–9)

According to this guidance it is evident that a doctor's primary duty in rela-tion to spiritual care is a medical duty of symptom control which may permit the patient to discuss spiritual concerns, although this is within an unassigned responsibility to elicit the patient's spiritual needs. The doctor is charged with recognizing that patients do consider spiritual matters, responding to them sympathetically and referring a seriously ill patient to a chaplain, priest or rabbi. The apologetic presumption is that few patients will raise spiritual issues directly with a doctor, but when they do so the doctor has a prescribed duty to ensure that the patient's world-view is respected. Twycross and Lack describe something of the doctor's duty in spiritual care in terms of both actions and omissions. In addition they suggest the limits of the responsibility assigned and some of the people whom the doctor may involve in discharg-ing other aspects of the obligation to provide for patients' spiritual needs.

In this scheme the doctor is to be aware of spiritual needs but refrain from discussing them unless the discussion is initiated by the patient. This argument is applied to few other aspects of a patient's needs, even when respect for patient autonomy is taken into account, and it is more remark-able because it is understood that most patients have need of 'spiritual help'. The omission of spirituality from the process of assessment inevitably diminishes the presence of this domain from considerations of care and the mobilization of resources. This applies equally to nurses who, for example through the admission and ongoing evaluation of patients, identify needs and plan interventions to address them. The overall presumption is that spiritual care is taking place by default, which provides all but the most tenuous assurance on the evidence presented. It also attests to the idea that spiritual care is absorbed in a general approach to care that simply 'happens' in palliative care because it is contained within its philosophy.

Uncertainty about spirituality both personally and professionally, a reluct-ance to appear ignorant or incompetent among peers, and the risk of self-disclosure may deflect a team from working towards a congruent approach to spiritual care and from clarifying roles and duties. Spirituality is a chal-lenge to the processes of care, but it may also represent a considerable individual threat because it is the locus for profound questions that are unavoidable in the face of suffering and death. Cornette (1997), reporting on a large-scale empirical study in Belgium among palliative care health-workers, remarks that:

> The reality is that, in the face of death, professional masks and uniforms tend to slip and questions about the meaning of life and death are stealing in upon all disciplines of caregivers. As long as this reality is denied, caregivers will never be able to listen to the full depth of each other's experiences and expectations. This appears to be a factor that may affect or erode patient care in the long run.
>
> (Cornette 1997: 11)

Figure 4.1 Providing spiritual care: a framework for inquiry

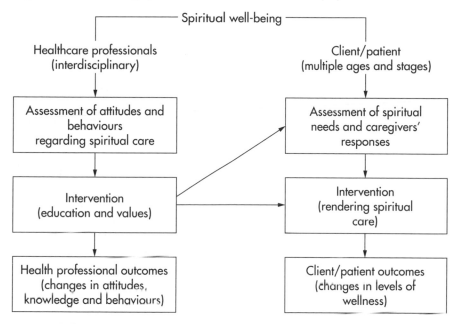

Source: Clark et al. 1991: 71

The ideal of the care team providing mutual support and enabling personal growth would appear to be compromised when the issue is spirituality. This may be explained by a sensitivity to respect the privacy of the individual, the absence of opportunities which allow spirituality to be 'safely' explored or a concern that admitting to having spiritual needs may be regarded as a weakness. It appears that it is acceptable for the sick to have spiritual needs but not their professional carers, and consequently this may desensitize those who work in palliative care to the spiritual domain.

A dichotomy between the philosophy and practice of palliative care is manifest in the domain of spiritual care when examined from the perspective of roles and responsibilities. Traditional religious aspects of care are generally much 'safer' for a team because they are well defined and the task can usually be assigned to a person with a specific office and responsibility. The ambiguity of spiritual care, compounded by the factors discussed, lend it to mystification or neglect and consequently a team may ostracize this aspect of care. Rather than its being integral to holism, spirituality becomes a peripheral consideration and practice.

An interdisciplinary approach provides a useful means of developing enhanced and integrated spiritual care (see Figure 4.1). The premise of the model is the interaction between patients and their professional carers that takes account of the knowledge, perceptions and actions of healthcare professionals. In other fields, practitioner formation, convention, training and accepted procedures clarify and promote duties, accountability and a consistent approach. This is generally not the case for spiritual care because perceived ambiguity limits operational practice. By addressing these factors through an interdisciplinary process the model anticipates that spiritual care will be clarified for the team in a way that is consistent with patients' needs. This requires individual team members to examine their own perspective on spirituality, and their own resources in responding to spiritual need. This then provides the basis for planning interventions for healthcare professionals that will enable them to improve the spiritual aspect of care.

This chapter has focused on the people who are involved in spiritual care and has provided a reflection on the reality as well as on the ideals. What we have not accounted for so far is the context within which this takes place: a context of both a culture with a distinct philosophy of care and a culture of a modern managed organization. It is these issues which also impact upon spirituality, shape its practice and must be equally open to critical reflection.

5 | The place of spirituality in palliative care

Palliative care has been a pioneering movement that has pushed out the boundaries of health care through developing innovative approaches to patient care and by promoting new attitudes and practices to dying and death now established in a distinct specialism. This creative work has promoted a set of goals and principles which have supported a multidisciplinary and multidimensional approach to care which has aimed to make central the interests of the patient. Related to these developments, palliative care has formed a distinctive culture or world-view that has been driven by a powerful, inspiring and essentially hopeful philosophy. Spirituality is a basic assumption in the palliative care narrative, and one which has been foundational to the modern hospice movement. In its evolution, palliative care has restated its belief in spiritual care, but in its practice it often appears to have become dislocated and problematic in relation to this philosophy. The place of spirituality in palliative care is revealing, therefore, of wider cultural influences, the effects of the way that health care is organized and the development of healthcare disciplines and professions. It is also inevitably a mirror reflecting the contemporary experiences and expressions of what it means to die, and therefore what it means to be human.

Spiritual care is one of the defining and distinctive principles of palliative care, but in many ways it remains one of the least developed and least explored aspects of the service. It may be argued that the spiritual dimension transcends the temporal, ever-changing world of health care and therefore remains in essence the same. But unless spirituality is to be banished to a hidden, inaccessible realm, it will remain enmeshed within the constraints and flux of our physical world. Similarly, spiritual care must be embodied and therefore subject to the implications of resource allocations, the complexities of human interaction and the capabilities of individual caregivers.

This pragmatic perspective on spiritual care locates spirituality within a service framework which is problematic as it tends towards a narrow, focused approach, whereas spirituality is expansive and always pointing beyond immediate limits. However, without some framework, some purposeful approach, spiritual care is likely to be a vague notion whose relationship to palliative care may become increasingly tangential.

Is spirituality intrinsic to palliative care?

Spirituality forms part of the vocabulary of palliative care, but as we explored in the previous chapter, its non-conformity to conventional processes of care and its ambiguity may leave spiritual care both unaccounted for in the discourse of organizational objectives and without a practical response. The assumption that the spiritual dimension is integral to palliative care philosophy is one that is largely unquestioned even though it is rarely explicated. While the philosophy of care may be regarded as sufficiently abstract to remain out of view of clinical practice it nevertheless guides the principles and foci of care and therefore has a tacit significance.

The aim of palliative care is to promote the well-being of patients in order to enhance their quality of life. This implies minimizing those things which impede, and maximizing those things which advance, a patient's best interests. In a healthcare setting it is generally understood that this aim is achieved by bringing about the patient's medical good. Randall and Downie (1996: 13–23) argue that as palliative care is an integral part of effective health care, its intrinsic aim is also that of the medical good:

> We shall maintain that in palliative care, as in the rest of health care, the intrinsic aim is to bring about what we shall call a 'medical good'. The term 'medical good' can never be precisely or completely analysed but we are using it as a blanket term to cover medical treatments such as those which lead to the amelioration or sometimes cure of disease processes, the relief of suffering, the prolongation of life, the dressing of wounds or injuries or many others. It is a characteristic feature of the treatments which lead to this 'medical good' that they are brought about by the use of drugs or technical procedures.
>
> (Randall and Downie 1996: 14)

Any non-medical good, they claim, is 'extrinsic' to the aim of health care because primarily there is no professional expertise or knowledge base which can qualify a carer to deal with spiritual and psychosocial matters other than practical wisdom. Training can be given to carers to advance the medical good, but it is life experience which is exercised in advancing the total good of the patient and which forms the mediator of technical skills.

There is an intimation in this argument that medical treatments can be considered in effective isolation from the other dimensions of personhood and that achieving the medical good relies upon effective technique alone. But the science of medicine cannot perceive the person, only recognize pathology, and it is with this incomplete knowledge that a doctor as a person has to establish a therapeutic relationship of trust and cooperation with the patient. A medical intervention aimed at bringing about a medical good cannot exclude the person of either the doctor or the patient. Medical expertise and knowledge, however convincing, have to be applied to the particular and the doctor must therefore have regard for the human being in totality. This is where the 'art' and 'science' of medicine must converge and the skills and abilities of the doctor are brought to the service rather than the manipulation of the patient.

It is undeniably the case that there is much at stake in what takes place between a doctor and patient and that this should attract the greatest moral consideration because life is generally regarded as being supremely valuable, significant and inviolable. Biological existence provides the foundation of life which is the basis for being human and being regarded as a person. But life as we understand it does not stop there: it takes on a broader meaning and purpose because we experience and express life through more than biology. In the field of terminal care, in particular, a healthy life is clearly a relative and not absolute value to the patient, even though it may be a primary value in the doctor/patient relationship. The medical good, for the patient, may even be considered an extrinsic value when assessed in the context of their overall aims. It is therefore much more than the crude manipulation of flesh and blood that we expect from doctors:

> The aim of medicine is to address not only the bodily assault that disease or injury inflicts but also the psychological, social, even spiritual dimensions of the assault. To heal is to make whole or sound . . .
>
> (Pellegrino and Thomasma 1988: 10)

Palliative care recognizes that medicine contributes in part to a patient's well-being. The precedence of medicine in palliative care cannot be ignored but nor should it be inflated. If the focus of palliative care is the promotion of the patient's best interests, then this is a goal to which more than medical interventions can be expected to contribute. The doctor has a distinct role to use medicine for the patient's good. However, a medical intervention, whilst achieving a recognized medical good or interest, may not be considered good by a patient whose centrality is such a feature of palliative care philosophy. The anxious patient will make a subjective judgement that may, for example, consider it preferable to see the chaplain in the context of a dedicated session than perhaps contemplate taking yet another quantity of tablets handed out by a hard-pressed nurse on a drugs round. It is hard to deny the purchase the medical profession and clinical science has on most people concerning treatment options, but this should not blind us to the ambiguities of medical interventions, not least for the terminally ill.

The different interpretations of the patient's good arise from the difference of interests of the various parties involved, but in palliative care it is the patient's best interests which are given priority and are usually encouraged. It is within this analysis that spiritual care should be considered. Pellegrino and Thomasma argue that the patient's good subsides in four aspects which operate concurrently and are interrelated: the patient's 'ultimate good', the good arising out of the freedom to choose, the patient's best interests and the medical good. The 'ultimate good' is the 'most pervasive, the least negotiable, and often the least explicit presupposition' (1988: 78) and it provides the reference standard against which choices are in the end arbitrated. This is the good that derives from a person's understanding of the ultimate purpose and destiny of human life and as such involves an individual's world-view, beliefs and faith. The good that derives from the capacity to choose is familiar in the principle of autonomy which Gillon (1985) summarizes as 'the capacity to think, decide, and act on the basis of such thought and decision freely and independently and without, as it says in the British passport, let or hindrance' (1985: 60). In palliative care the promotion of a patient's autonomy is taken as a primary consideration in order that a patient may shape the course of their living and dying, even in ways which to others may be considered irrational, unwise or simply wrong. Through exercising choice, people can strive to live in a way that is consistent with their understanding of the ultimate good; it expresses beliefs and creates meaning according to what they consider to be in their best interest. Finally in this scheme, we take account of the medical good which encompasses the treatment of disease and symptom control. As Pellegrino and Thomasma contend, 'There always is an unfortunate tendency for physicians to equate biomedical good with the whole of the patient's good . . . Biomedical good does not exhaust the good the physician is obliged to do. It is an essential but not sufficient component of good medicine' (1988: 78).

What else is counted as essential is a contentious question in a resource-limited service, but priorities have to be allocated, and interests have to be negotiated. It is in this practical and particular context that the philosophy of palliative care has to work, and it is in this context that spiritual care is afforded time, space and personnel. It is also in this context that we have to consider the ethical question of what *should* palliative care consist of. The analysis in which we have considered the aim of palliative care demonstrates that it is much wider than a physical good and that the patient's good prevails wherever possible. Spiritual care, alongside medical care, can contribute to the patient's good, and for the patient that which supports and fosters their ultimate purpose and destiny – their spiritual orientation – may be considered as much an intrinsic aim of palliative care as a medical good. Randall and Downie (1996) maintain that a commitment to the relief of suffering underpins the ethos of palliative care. Whilst they recognize that there are many factors related to wholeness, 'however much we may want to influence all these other factors we must accept that there are necessary practical and philosophical limits to the scope of professional activity in palliative care' (Randall and Downie 1996: 152). We have dealt with some of these limits, but we need to attend further to the ethical nature of spiritual care.

Spiritual care, like the practice of medicine, cannot be considered as an independent moral action separate from the wider frame of the patient's interests. It is unlikely that most spiritual care practices can be regarded as a trespass against the person, but even if a practice may of itself be considered benign, if it is imposed upon a patient, if it contravenes a patient's beliefs, if it disrupts the aims and plans of a patient, it may not be considered beneficent unless a stronger argument for paternalism is invoked. Equally, although patient autonomy is impeded by illness, this does not obligate carers to fulfil patient's interests without any consideration of either what is good or of the wider interests of society. There is therefore the need for the patient and the carer to be engaged in an ethical relationship in which a dialogue can be developed, driven by the goal of the patient's good.

The patient/carer dialogue and the resulting course of action are traditionally shaped by the medical profession in health care with its emphasis on the biomedical model of disease. In palliative care a broader perspective allows the dialogue to be influenced by other disciplines, to engage with components of the patient's good beyond the medical, and to incorporate a patient-orientated view of illness. This is not intended to undervalue the medical contribution or to discount the role of the doctor as a person in the therapeutic encounter, but it does demonstrate an approach that seeks to address the needs of a person as a whole including spiritual needs. However, there is some debate as to whether there is a retrograde trend in palliative care towards medicalization with its emphasis on malfunction and pathology. This shift away from the whole person has consequences not only for the nature of the care offered but also for the ethical relationship. Corner and Dunlop (1997), in reflecting upon the development of palliative care, surmise that, 'The biomedical understanding is felt to be profoundly limiting of healing in its broadest sense and has contributed to the development of the counter-cultures of consumerism and alternative models of healing' (Corner and Dunlop 1997: 292).

The patient/carer relationship is intersected by discourses of healing and well-being that are central to the existential and spiritual concerns of what it means to be human and which draw upon many different perspectives and understandings. But we must note another limit, and that is the palliative care setting itself which delineates acceptable care and hermeneutics. Palliative care, for example, does not tolerate the absolute exercise of patient autonomy: euthanasia is not regarded as an acceptable course of action. Nor does it count all interpretations of dying valid or equal: a patient dying in pain is likely to be regarded as less good. There is therefore a *modus vivendi* of palliative care that requires both patient and health carers to work within a certain context of practice, morality and spirituality typi- fied, for example, by the much criticized notion of a good death. Within this, non-medical interventions have been both a challenge and a conces- sion to the dynamics of power between the public and the professions. But if palliative care is committed to promoting the best interests of patients then spiritual care must be more than tolerated, it must also be part of the ethical relationship. This requires that such spiritual care practices are examined with the rigour demonstrated by the medical precedent and practised with an equal regard to the rights, duties and responsibilities that establish and govern the patient/carer relationship.

The organization of spirituality

Contemporary palliative care services, unlike their ancient predecessors, are subject as much to developments in management theory as they are to therapeutic innovations. The National Health Service and voluntary sector have been greatly influenced by systems, usually originating in manufactur- ing industry, which aim to maximize output and profit through effective and efficient processes and people. The shift from the administration to the management of health services is evident in, for example, the drive for 'quality' which originates in an industrial objective that has been success- fully translated into health care and is becoming an important indicator of 'performance'. In this section, therefore, we consider spiritual care as an aspect of the contemporary organization of palliative care services. The critique will follow some of the analysis of managed organizations sug- gested by Pattison (1997).

One of the reasons that the modern hospice movement has been so suc- cessful is its inspiring vision that is basically concerned with promoting a better way to die. The utopian aspect of this vision has already been noted, but its appeal rests upon a strong sense that people facing a terminal illness, which could one day be any of us, should be afforded the best care avail- able in the nicest environment and every effort made to maximize quality of life. It is a vision which has motivated people highly because of its instinc- tual moral appeal and its comforting compensation for the grim prospects that dying and death hold for many. It is a modern vision of *the art of dying* in which spirituality has become an aspect of this ideal representing the 'mystical' fourth dimension of care and accommodating the concerns many have about their ultimate destiny. In the hospice movement this has been captured in the use of religious imagery and nomenclature, but in general a sense of compassion and peacefulness is communicated in the vision that suggests that hospice and palliative care are sacred, venerable and possibly the next best thing to godliness.

The palliative care ideal has been extremely effective in persuading people and mobilizing resources, but its realization has been limited to a small number of services dealing with particular categories of illness. This is not to belittle the impact this has made upon the care of the terminally ill in general, but it does indicate that one of the inevitable consequences of idealism is expectations that can be greatly beyond the reach of the reality. Most people would prefer to die at home but will die in hospital, and in the study by Dunlop et al. (1989), of the 29 per cent who expressed a preference to die in a hospice, only 12 per cent actually did. There are many intervening factors to explain some of this gap, and it would be wrong to suppose that hospital is necessarily a worse place to die, but a problem with idealism is that it generates simplistic contrasts and stimulates unmet demand:

Presently, users and service providers are caught up in colluding to idealize public services. Encouraged by managerial and political rhetoric, users feel that services are a kind of omniproviding parent that should respond immediately to their every need, however unreasonable. Providers aspire to unbounded parental providence, feeling unable to be honest and say openly that some services cannot be provided, or not in the way or to the extent that users might like.

(Pattison 1997: 83)

The spiritual dimension of palliative care in its ideal form is the final piece of the holistic jigsaw completing the integrated whole. The disciplines involved in palliative care feel that they must in some way contribute to this dimension and extend their scope of responsibility to ensure that they are obligated to respond to this need. This generates expectations that spirituality will be within the professional grasp, that spiritual care can be attainable by all with the sufficient training and skills, and that spiritual needs whatever they are can be satisfied. But the ideal of spirituality ensures that it can never be reached, for this level of perfection can be realized only in ideology, not in reality. The ideal also suggests that anything is possible in spiritual care, there appear to be no limits or compromises:

To be a chaplain in a highly charged emotional environment, such as a hospice sometimes is, one must be something of a dancing chameleon, taking on the colour and shading of others' worlds, able to move lightly into and out of the linguistic modes of doctors and nurses, of patients, with their varying backgrounds, upbringing and occupational training, and the loved ones of those patients, the varying dynamics of relational networks. By body language, by tone of voice, by the sensitivity to judge a moment – when to say nothing, when to touch, when to make a joke – by facial expression, a carer must communicate what should never be said; 'I understand.'

(Wilcock 1996: 47)

The simplification necessary for promoting an ideal vision requires that certain aspects of reality are excluded or even denied, and a consequence of this may be that self-criticism is dampened. When this vision is projected inwards onto the organization, it gives it a clarity of purpose that becomes its mission. An organization looking forward to achieving excellence is orientated on what is as yet unrealized and may devalue or undermine what is currently happening and the efforts put into delivering the service today. The past may also be of little significance in working towards what lies ahead, despite the reality that both palliative care and the charities and National Health Service which support it all have remarkable histories. Matters of life and death are constant companions of humankind and the legacy of human thought and imagination in dealing with their existence and destiny has been expressed in words and ideas that have much to say to us today. But the cutting-edge may be more valued than old knowledge which is deemed obsolete. Instead, change is inevitable and all things must be updated, including spiritual care which cannot rely upon relics from the past but must be upgraded and transformed.

Underpinning the mission of the organization are the objectives which can be translated into the tasks and processes necessary to achieve the vision. At an individual level, these objectives determine the roles within the organization and the skills required to perform them. Performance is the operative word in a managed organization for such organizations generally account for what is demonstrable and place value on what is obviously relevant to the mission. The spiritual aspect of care is therefore increasingly subject to attempts to make it conform to verifiable processes and measurable outcomes within a rationalized framework of knowledge and skills. A problem with this approach is that:

the kind of understanding and wisdom that comes from life and which may be very valuable in, say, caring relationships may be disregarded. Similarly, the tendency to break jobs and occupations down into analysable units may in fact distort the holistic nature of a job. Nurses, for example, protest that the performance of their job is more than applying atomized skills.

(Pattison 1997: 93)

Spiritual care reduced to another package of training or discrete technique will fail to incorporate much of the breadth and depth which the spiritual dimension concerns. Narrowing spirituality to something that can be neatly dealt with by fulfilling a specified task may enable it to find a place within the managed organization but it is unlikely that it will be able to deal with the messy unpredictability of human beings. This applies similarly to the drive to measure outcomes which relies upon having the 'apparatus' to make the measurement and an accepted set of quantifiable values. Interventions can then be systematically evaluated for their effectiveness, but the simplicity of this theory belies its difficulties, for what at first seems to offer precision may founder upon the ambiguities of multifaceted factors and the innumerable variables involved.

Happiness is a good example. What is meant by happiness? Is it a mental state of euphoria and intoxication? Is it a physiological state of satiability in all senses? Is it a matter of having the needs of human existence, such as nutrition and shelter, satisfied? Or does happiness concern human desires and dreams being fulfilled? For the theory to be effective there must be some attempt at an objective notion of happiness, a standard that is beyond individual taste and value. The theory relies on the presumption that most people understand happiness in a consistent and self-evident manner. Assuming that happiness means the same to all people at all times, can it be measured, or assigned a value? Without this the theory cannot be used to assess the effects of the action. Clearly, if happiness is measured by reference to objective means, such as the number of wins on the lottery, this can be used to provide a valid and reliable score: valid in the sense that it measures what is intended, and reliable in the sense that it is consistent across many measurements. However, if happiness relies upon more abstract means, and particularly those that refer to quality, some form of interpretation and representation will need to take place before a value can be placed upon them, which may reduce their objectivity, reliability and validity.

The attempts at measuring spiritual well-being can be readily criticized for their imprecision and weak validity and reliability. But in palliative care, if something is not measurable will it be devalued or perhaps become unrecognized? Considering that the spiritual domain includes much that is elusive, it will consistently fail the utilitarian test despite its possible significance and value to an individual or palliative care service. A service focused on outcomes may therefore 'displace thinking about wider factors that might be highly pertinent, particularly in organizations that deliver services to other human beings which of their very nature must have elements of process, subjectivity, unpredictability and intangibility' (Pattison 1997: 95). This is not to suggest that spiritual care should be exempted from questions of purpose, benefit or cost, but it is to question whether the notion of care accounted for by outcomes may consequently lead to significant aspects of human experience being abandoned because they lie outside the limited confines of business management.

The modern managed palliative care service undoubtedly offers good care and can demonstrate improvements on its predecessors' efforts. In

adopting the assumptions, theories and practices of performance and pro-
ductivity, services have sought to demonstrate their effectiveness and relevance to health care and wider society. There is an inherent tension in this
position because palliative care arose out of a radical critique of certain
postwar norms and practices but aimed to be accepted and supported by
the very same community.

This process of assimilation may be no less evident with regard to the
concept of spirituality which has undergone a major shift from its original
position. The religious foundation of the modern hospice movement,
exemplified in St Christopher's Hospice, translated a theological basis for
the care of the terminally ill into a modern scientific healthcare context.
Bradshaw (1996b) suggests that Cicely Saunders, originator of the modern
hospice movement, revived a tradition for the dying that Florence Nightingale had established for nursing, namely a spiritual ethic of care that was
rooted in Christian faith. But palliative care became increasingly subject to
the process of secularization in which spirituality referred less to God and
more to humanity, so that religious beliefs and values were superseded by
'expert' skills and knowledge. Secularization, laments Bradshaw, 'appears
to be the process by which palliative care no longer acknowledges or indeed
has any place for its traditional spiritual conscience. It has been replaced by
secularizing ideas from the psychological and social sciences' (Bradshaw
1996b: 418). Palliative care rationalized in this way is no longer at the
service of a more 'ultimate' purpose but becomes an end in itself.

In tracing the evolution of the theories and practices of spiritual care
Walter (1997) identifies three approaches taken in palliative care. The first
approach is that of the religious community in which faith matters and
preparing for death is preparing for the life beyond death. Hospices with
Christian foundations and those which explicitly include faith practices
still exist but it is hard to find examples of palliative care services that
can be described as religious communities. The second response to
spiritual issues is exemplified by referring patients to a chaplain. In this
approach there is no distinction of the spiritual from the religious and it is
only the clergy who are regarded as capable of dealing with this domain.
As Walter remarks, it has the advantage that spiritual care can easily be
assigned to the chaplain but it is an approach which is incompatible with
the notion of holistic care that is widespread in palliative care. In the
third approach, by contrast, spiritual care becomes the responsibility of the
multidisciplinary team because it concerns the human search for meaning
which is applicable to everyone regardless of faith. This concept of spirituality effectively fulfils the holistic aims of palliative care and 'squares the
otherwise unsquareable circle of how to provide spiritual care for all patients in a secular setting' (Walter 1997: 26). As we have seen, however, this
widely adopted approach is not without problems, and despite the apparent prosperity of spirituality evident in the discourses of palliative care,

spirituality's conformity to secular systems may also be the root of the discontent discussed by Bradshaw.

In this section we have taken a deliberately critical view of the organizational developments of palliative care in relation to the changes that have affected spiritual care. The intention has not been to support an organizational Luddism or to rehabilitate some 'golden era' of spiritual care. It is a proper obligation of palliative care that it should strive to make good use of its share of resources; that it should aim to ensure that its practices are beneficial; that it should explore new approaches. Palliative care does not operate in a sacrosanct space even though it may be regarded as occupying 'holy' ground. Similarly, spiritual care, however conceived, is rooted in a particular context involving practical, ethical, theological and social considerations. It diminishes any aspect of care to treat it as just an abstract function, for spiritual care is not simply a process any more than palliative care is simply technique. Therefore the assumptions of contemporary healthcare management need to be taken with caution, because its utilitarian solutions do not remove the ambiguities and complexities that face us in life and in death.

New directions in spiritual care

In considering the place of spirituality in palliative care we have focused mostly upon the type of established institutional 'specialist' services that developed out of the hospice model. Palliative care has become an increasingly mobile philosophy whose itinerant course is evident through the spread of the 'palliative care approach' in increasingly diverse settings. The spiritual care of the hospice movement has not been left behind and it is therefore emerging in new contexts and places. In this final section we visit a number of areas which suggest new directions for spiritual care. In doing so we shall look at the problems which this may present and outline some of the potential benefits which it may bring.

Hospital palliative care

the *real* event taking place at the end of our life is our death, not the attempts to prevent it. We have somehow been so taken up with the wonders of modern science that our society puts the emphasis in the wrong place. It is the dying that is the important thing – the central player in the drama is the dying man; the dashing leader of that bustling squad of his would-be rescuers is only a spectator, and a groundling at that.

(Nuland 1994: 256)

If grim experiences of dying in hospital were a major impetus to the foundation of the modern hospice movement then it is in a return to hospitals that palliative care finds an appropriate location. The experience and expertise developed in specialist units have become translated primarily into nurse-led teams who provide advice and support to hospital staff, patients and those significant to them. In addition there is a growing involvement of palliative care from the point of diagnosis through joint outpatient clinics. The mechanism for involving a member of the palliative care team for an in-patient usually requires the consent of the admitting consultant to a request from ward-based staff. In responding to a referral the team member is likely to carry out a full assessment and apply an holistic framework. This introduces the spiritual aspect and may involve some formal assessment in addition to the interpretation of the patient and carer narratives (Glickman 1996).

Hospitals are not devoid of the spiritual aspects of care, and since its inception the National Health Service has officially made provision for spiritual care in the form of chaplaincies. Chaplains in hospitals are spread out far more thinly than they are in specialist units, and in acute hospitals may operate mainly through prioritized referrals. In large hospitals the demands of, for example, critical care, trauma and maternity wards may occupy significant although unpredictable amounts of time, further limiting chaplains' availability to meet less specified needs. Hospital chaplaincies are usually expected to function principally in the mode of religious representatives for patients requesting pastoral care specific to a faith community, and this is customarily how their number is determined. However, hospital chaplains may make less of the distinction between the religious and the spiritual and may be well versed in the philosophy of holistic care.

A problem facing a hospital palliative care service in all its aspects is that it is only a guest on someone else's territory. The purpose of most acute care remains the management of disease, restorative interventions and active treatment so that the inclusion of palliative care from the point of life-threatening diagnosis remains remote for many patients with non-malignant disease. Consequently, the perception and permitted practice of palliative care may be one that is compressed into later stages of disease progression, when symptoms are less responsive. These constraints shape the notion of spiritual care that can be realized for a patient so that the spiritual aspect may be associated more with dying than with living. As with other aspects of care, the palliative care representative will have to negotiate the adoption of spiritual care recommendations or the involvement of a palliative care chaplain. Issues of jurisdiction, intraprofessional relationships and limited resources may become some of the other factors that mediate this involvement.

Hospital palliative care extends from clinical work to include education and training. This provides a forum for the spiritual aspects of the palliative care approach to be promoted and instilled in acute care staff as part of the holistic philosophy. It may encourage ward staff to practise the palliative model of spiritual care and to involve members of the palliative care team when spiritual needs have been identified. Acute care, however, is not a desert in terms of spiritual aspects of care and it is beneficial for palliative care staff to engage with the experiences of staff in this context. As a peripatetic service, hospital palliative care will always rely upon the relationships it establishes with the wards to which it is invited. The challenge to the palliative care team is how to ensure that spiritual aspects of care are given the same attention as symptom control and that ward staff incorporate their recommendations into the care plan.

Community care

> The solitary death is now so well recognized that our society has organized against it, and well we should. From the wisdom of the legal documents called advanced directives to the questionable philosophies of suicide societies, a range of options exists, and at bottom the goal of each of them is the same: a restoration of certainty that when the end is near, there will be at least this source of hope – that our last moments will be guided not by the bioengineers but by those who know who we are.
>
> (Nuland 1994: 255)

Care routes for people with terminal illness typically involve a combination of sites and these will include the domiciliary setting with its related services as well as 'community' hospitals, satellite day care units, and residential and nursing homes. The development of community palliative care has been closely related to growth in numbers of Macmillan nurses, Marie Curie nurses and home support teams alongside general practitioners and district nurses. A substantial aspect of domiciliary orientated services involves symptom control and interventions aimed at supporting patients and those who care for them in their community. There is little evidence that spiritual care has been considered in this setting. In a specialist care unit, a number of disciplines may contribute to the provision of spiritual care and there will usually be access to some chaplaincy provision. In a community setting, the provision may be less coordinated and concurrent with very restricted access to chaplaincy. Local faith communities may offer some form of provision, but the level of provision will depend upon the patient's location, faith affiliation and previous association. Primary care staff may neither have developed any particular skills in assessing spiritual care needs nor have effective mechanisms for referrals. However, more than their hospital counterparts, health professionals in domiciliary settings usually have better privacy and patients may feel more able to talk on their own home ground.

As a patient passes from different settings in the course of their illness and treatment path there will be inevitable and expected variations in the level and form of spiritual care available. The relationship between sites of care and the provision of services composes a complex process, but much will depend upon the effectiveness of communication and the comparability of resources. Spiritual care may be subject to fragmentation and discontinuity or be ill-considered in a care setting whose philosophy is predominantly physically orientated. Specialist palliative care services are typically an adjunct to community services but contend that, as a philosophy, and not a place of care, it can be applied and delivered wherever the patient resides. How this is realized for the spiritual aspects of care is rarely expounded by services and it is unclear where the responsibility rests. Equally, there are no empirical data to suggest what the need for such a service may be.

At present there is no established service provision for consistent and accessible spiritual care that covers community settings. A limited service may be offered by community services and the community-based work of palliative care professionals. If a service need is determined then one approach is suggested by community mental health services: a community palliative care chaplain. The key purpose of this role would be the provision of spiritual care across domiciliary and community settings that is integrated within the overall package of care. Such a chaplain would offer:

• spiritual care for community-based patients;
• liaison and consultation with the care team and sites of care;
• referral to local faith communities when appropriate;
• training opportunities and consultation for faith community representatives, community professionals and community groups;
• a professional and accountable service.

The development of a strategy for community chaplaincy will need to take account of existing structures of palliative care provision and community care. The strategy will need to be unambiguous and clear in defining the role of the community chaplain so that it is consistent with the objectives of community services and respectful of the care offered by community-based organizations, religious and otherwise. Community chaplaincy raises many questions for which a feasibility study would be beneficial. The study would assess the level of need as well as the practical implementation of such a service. The funding of such a post, its management and operation would all be issues to clarify, but existing models for other professional services may provide an initial framework which can be adapted.

Different faiths

When I have a major illness requiring highly specialized treatment, I will seek out a doctor skilled in its provision. But I will not expect of him that he understand my values, my expectations for myself and those I love, my spiritual nature, or my philosophy of life. That is not what he is trained for and that is not what he will be good at. It is not what drives those engines of excellence.

(Nuland 1994: 266)

Spirituality and spiritual care in the context of Euro-American palliative care are predominantly concepts that developed out of a Christian tradition in which the modern hospice movement was located. When we consider different faith traditions we encounter different world-views (see Chapter 2) and accounts of spirituality to the extent that the word itself may be unknown. The meaning of illness, the nature of suffering and humankind's ultimate destiny may be aspects of a particular spirituality that delineate it from other accounts. Here we encounter spirituality in a context which has acquired sociocultural details that distinguish it from a general humanist account. Contextualized spirituality takes account of interrelated aspects such as beliefs, ethics and rituals which contribute to diverse spiritual expressions and experiences. Any attempt to uphold spirituality as a global concept depends therefore upon its being understood either as the lowest common human denominator or a term providing a 'sacred canopy' under which to gather diverse spiritual traditions. In either approach it is the details provided by the patient narratives which inform staff and guide the provision of spiritual care.

Voluntary and National Health Service palliative care services in the UK do not take an impartial approach to spiritual care: such care may be an explicitly religious, nominally Christian, secularized Christian or a humanist account which operates at an organizational level and will be evident in such things as the processes of care, the types of staff employed and the facilities available. Respect for patient autonomy means that services have to be responsive to the spiritual needs arising from different faith and cultural traditions. In particular, staff need to be able to explore with a patient what spirituality means to them in a broad and dynamic sense and not simply in reduced terms of, for example, dietary requirements or faith practices. The perspective of contextualized spirituality may question received practice, knowledge and the professional and organizational status of a service claiming to encompass spiritual care. This takes spirituality out of the benign mould into which it is often placed and opens it to being something more kaleidoscopic, creative and challenging. An assumption that theism is the norm, for example, will not only be irrelevant to a follower of Jainism (Bowker 1997: 487–8) but may well obscure important aspects of the person's spiritual orientation and their care needs.

The disproportionate number of people using hospice and specialist palliative care services from the black and ethnic minority communities has received some attention in the literature (Hill and Penso 1997; Smaje and

Field 1997) but these do not provide an extensive treatment of the many faiths present in the population. Whatever the proportion of people from different faith communities using palliative care services, a number of questions present themselves: how accessible and involved are representatives from these communities in informing the service about spiritual issues, in planning service developments, in staff training and in the provision of spiritual care? It is usually the task of the (Christian) chaplain to coordinate referrals for spiritual care outside of the care team, and the success of this will depend upon how established and effective links are with the wider communities. However, people from different faith communities must not have their spiritual care isolated to a visiting minister any more than it should be directed by information contained in a folder labelled 'special needs'. Spiritual care, rather than being isolated to discrete practices and interventions, needs to be integrated into the many interfaces between the person and the service. There needs to be a self-awareness by staff of the assumptions and world-view with which they frame their own experiences and by which they perceive the experiences and behaviour of others.

Professionals encountering people of different faiths may feel threatened as much as intrigued; equally patients may be disquieted by attitudes and assumptions expressed through individuals and the practices and procedures of a service. It is through engaging with difference that a service may better understand its own philosophy and ideology and the way these inform its practice. This may enable professionals to explore more openly the spiritual dimension of care and understand more clearly the way in which their own spiritual orientations are involved. In a rare example of a palliative care service established upon the principles of a Buddhist philosophy, McGrath (1998) reports upon how this explicit spiritual orientation contributes to defining the service in which the spiritual 'ideology' of both the hospice and Buddhist discourses (Mahayana tradition) combine in the commitment to caring for the dying. In particular, Buddhist notions of compassion and wisdom, the importance of a practical metaphysic, a willingness to serve, tolerance, the duty to do no harm, and the significance of death are seen as commensurable with and supportive of hospice practice (McGrath 1998: 260).

People with non-cancer diagnoses

Nature has a job to do. It does its job by the method that seems most suited to each individual whom its powers have created. It has made this one susceptible to heart disease and that one to stroke and yet another to cancer, some after a long time on this earth and some after a time much too brief, at least by our own reckoning.

(Nuland 1994: 262)

There is a cautiously extending list of mortal illnesses which are considered suitable for palliative care. The addition to cancer of diagnoses which may benefit from a similar approach is not without contention. The legacy of support for cancer care pulls in one direction and the ethical argument of justice pulls in the other. In 1982 a man died from a condition whose viral origins had to wait another year to be identified and a further four years to be officially named: human immunodeficiency virus, HIV. The man was called Terrence Higgins, and his lover and friends formed a trust to establish a service for people living with and affected by AIDS. Subsequently, community and in-patient services were developed specifically to respond to what was believed at the time to be an epidemic that would become the greatest mortal disease in the UK. HIV-related disease and AIDS presented many challenges to health services, not least in terms of the availability and accessibility of palliative care. The controversy of cancer-dedicated services accepting non-cancer patients is now not limited to AIDS. Patients with other life-threatening diseases, such as terminal cardiac failure or chronic respiratory diseases are challenging the compass of palliative care services whose philosophy of care can without difficulty be applied to a wide range of fatal diseases.

When we consider the spiritual aspect of care for people with diagnoses other than cancer we find general similarities but also distinct differences. The way a progressive condition develops, the manifestation and combination of specific symptoms, its incursions into life and the approach to death may result in diverse aspects of terminal illness. Diseases, whatever clinically they may represent, are also social constructions and acquire their own distinct metaphors, meanings, values, morality, politics and expectations. Perspectives such as these condition the personal experience of being ill and represent a disease narrative that informs the individual's perception. These many factors impress upon the spiritual aspects of living with a terminal diagnosis which for non-cancer diseases may raise unparalleled issues. Motor neurone disease may be considered as one example of a non-malignant condition with spiritual implications that may result from living with progressive muscle weakness, the resulting quality of life, and the manner of death. Cardiac failure represents another condition characterized by a further set of spiritual issues with its temporal consequences, psychological sequelae, distressing symptoms and often suddenness of death (Gibbs et al. 1998: 961–2).

The spiritual care developed in a predominantly cancer context has much that it can bring to the palliative care of people with non-cancer diagnoses and there exists already some interaction between these two groups through hospital palliative care services and to a lesser extent specialist units. A simple replication of existing spiritual care may not provide the most appropriate or useful service. Patients, for example, in particular disease groups may take very different care pathways and this will determine the accessibility and continuity of services. This is another area where there is a paucity of research upon which to establish new practice, but the growing experience of palliative care in this widening field indicates that the spiritual aspects of care need attending to as much as any other.

The integration of different patient groups into a service accustomed to cancer will have implications greater than the availability of resources and the appropriateness of current care models. Spiritual care is one such area that will also need to learn from different perspectives and the experiences of patients whose biographies may present many new challenges. But through engaging with people whose diagnoses are less familiar to palliative care it may also become enriched:

> Through working with people with AIDS, I have discovered, to my surprise, a faith that runs very deep. Faith in a higher power certainly, and in the spark of that same power which exists in human beings – the power to fight for life, to struggle to realise our greatest potential, the power to live, dream and find moments of happiness against all odds, and the power it takes to surrender to the inevitable when the time is right.
>
> (Richman 1994: 37)

6 A professional approach to spiritual care

The doors fly open on a male surgical ward as a consultant and a train of junior doctors arrive for the ward round. The consultant heads straight for a particular bed where, surrounded by eager students, he exposes the patient's abdomen, draws a line across it indicating the place of incision, and addresses the students as to the nature of the surgery. Finally the consultant speaks to the now obviously distressed patient, 'Now don't worry, this has nothing whatsoever to do with you!' Sir Lancelot Spratt epitomized in the *Doctor* . . . films may have been the product of an imaginative scriptwriter, but he characterized the apparent disregard of patients in a time when few would dare to question such exalted professionals. The doctor knew best and did the best for his patient, that was the privilege of his professional status which attested to his recognized competence to perform, in this case, major invasive surgery.

Few would accept the attitude and practice of Sir Lancelot Spratt in this extreme form today because the balance between patients' autonomy and the beneficent paternalism of doctors has shifted considerably. The point of the illustration is to introduce some of the issues that surface around all healthcare actions which take place between a dependent patient and person who represents a discipline with the 'authority' to act in such a way that ordinarily would result in a crime or be regarded as abuse or damage of the person's interests. If spiritual care is to be realized it will involve the actions of certain people claiming competence that carries some potential risk of harm, even though they do not directly compromise a person's bodily integrity. In addition there is the general necessity in a place of care for patients to be able to put their trust in those who exercise roles which provide care. Few would oblige a stranger offering poisonous drugs as a treatment unless that person were a registered doctor suggesting chemotherapy. But that is the level of trust and risk we are prepared to take with medical personnel and to a lesser extent other healthcare disciplines. There is in effect a trade between competence and trust which not only helps to establish the fiduciary relationship but also paves the way for the consent that justifies the action. For spiritual care to happen, therefore, patients need to be reassured that by entering a therapeutic relationship for this purpose they will come to no harm, that they can trust in the people involved and that they have adequate information to accept or reject the proposed action.

There are a number of interrelated areas that we shall consider in this chapter, none of which is unique to spiritual care, because spiritual care cannot lie outside the moral compass of health care. More contentious, however, is whether spiritual care can be provided without training, assessment of competence and regulation of practice, for this leads us into the area of authority, rights and responsibilities. Patients ought to be protected from unskilled or unprincipled practitioners, and they ought to be able to rely upon a duty of care which is implicit in all actions and worthy of every confidence. If this ethical foundation were not present then palliative care users would be subject to arbitrary relationships with practitioners with uncertain grounds for trust. However, not all care practices carry the same moral implications and certain roles carry a greater moral responsibility because of the claims that practitioners make about their actions and motives. Therefore we shall consider spiritual care and its practice in the same register that all other aspects of palliative care are considered.

Professional practice

In the course of this book the term 'healthcare professional' has been used loosely to describe people who use a distinctive expertise or learning in their commitment to further the interests of patients for whom they care. The questions we explore in this section concern whether or not spiritual care warrants professional practice and who is a professional capable of providing spiritual care.

There is much contention as to who may be called a professional, but of interest to us is that the word has become the shorthand for someone whose practice is regarded as legitimate, of a high standard and to be valued. A common characteristic of a profession is the claim to some form of privilege and uniqueness for its membership over above that of the general public. The basis for the privilege lies traditionally in the unique expertise and actions of a professional undertaken on behalf of others. In essence, a healthcare professional is one who acts for the benefit or good of the patient and does so with sufficient competence, accountability, fidelity and discretion to justify being trusted (Koehn 1994). These conditions also provide the grounds for the authority and the legitimization of the particular role as well as its limits. In the case of doctors and clergy, this has found historical expression in the tradition of a public commitment – a literal profession. However, through membership, other disciplines affect this commitment by means of binding codes of conduct and public registration.

Professionals can therefore claim to be different from the general public in their commitment to serve a particular good and in the obligations that this entails. To accomplish this it is expected that professionals will have adequate training to perform their functions and duties. A specialist or technical knowledge historically not only conferred status to the individual but also provided the profession with a considerable degree of autonomy. However, it is not uncommon today to hear of doctors confronted by patients with information gained through the Internet concerning treatments that have yet to be published in respected medical publications. Similarly, there are many shelves in most bookshops dedicated to spirituality in its most diverse forms and no end of self-help guides to assist the troubled soul on its spiritual journey. But professional practice is not defined exclusively by expertise because the expert has no moral commitment to any other good apart from perfecting knowledge which may promote a self-interest. The professional is aware that this is not the only knowledge that must be considered, for there is the self-knowledge of individuals, including the conception of what is good, which must be respected and which allows the individual to refuse what the professional offers.

In palliative care it is a commitment to the patient's good which distinguishes the relationship between a professional and a member of the wider public, for it is a commitment in which the former's moral probity and competence are exchanged for the trust and particular interests of the latter. From this extends both a dependence of patients and the much criticized power which professionals claim and defend. A so-called expert on spirituality may provide a useful reference but has made no pledge to put this knowledge to the service of others. If there can be professionals who render spiritual care it will be in part because of their commitment to promote this aspect of the patient's good.

However, the goal of the relationship between the healthcare professional and the patient is far more ambiguous in palliative care than it is in more general health. The restoration of health is the fundamental and widely accepted profession of the physician, but the medical care of the dying represents what is, in essence, a modern development. What it means to die well is open to considerable discussion and different approaches. Appeals by palliative care to the promotion of well-being do not reduce this ambiguity and add yet further relative values. Chaplains, specifically, do not encounter this difficulty because dying and death do not undermine the good they promote, the patient's ultimate purpose and destiny. It is not necessary to further define this good – that will happen between the patient and the chaplain – but the point is that, like other goods which professionals promote, it is an end in itself and considered to be so by the wider public, hence the traditional goods of health, justice and salvation.

If spiritual care aims to contribute more than a general sense of well-being and its claim to deal with 'ultimate' matters is to be sanctioned then the relationship between patient and carer will require an ethical orientation that is based upon more than expertise, technique or good intentions. The professional ethic has traditionally provided the basis of the relationship in many faith communities, and this has transferred into health care in the form of chaplains. But, given that many patients have only a nominal relationship with a faith community, the legitimization of this role will be more than a matter of faith. Pellegrino and Thomasma (1988) argue that the ethical character of professional relationships is determined by specific duties: a public commitment to beneficence based upon competence, a mutual valuation of the intended goal, the fulfilment of role-specific duties and the promotion of moral agency (Pellegrino and Thomasma 1988: 66–8). In relation to spiritual care, several issues emerge. Is it a specific responsibility and a duty of a particular role (Chapter 4)? What constitutes the competence for spiritual care? And does it warrant its own distinct profession or can it be subsumed within existing professions?

In order to safeguard patients from the potential harm inherent in professional practices, patients need to be assured that the person to whom they are entrusting themselves is sufficiently skilled and knowledgeable that risks and bad consequences are minimized. Competence as a professional duty is not intended to imply a blanket guarantee for all matters dealt with, but is focused on defined areas. Competence is not extensive and a patient would be justifiably concerned with the claims, for example, that a competent chiropodist will therefore, by extension, be able to provide psychotherapy. Ensuring that the limitations of practitioners are well understood and maintained has a dual benefit in that it prescribes the areas which professionals may justifiably act and allows for patients to be informed about the limits of their expertise. Competence therefore maintains the integrity of both the professional and the patient, releasing the former from having to fulfil unrealistic demands and reassuring the latter that professional boundaries will be maintained.

Education and training is the normal route for a person to gain minimal professional competence (qualifications) which is then attached to the continual development of proficiency and ongoing learning (grade). This temporal dimension to competence is reflected in the career structures of professions and is alluded to in the titular hierarchy, the point being that competence for most professionals is not simply attained but acquired and developed over time. There is little evidence that healthcare professionals have attended to spiritual matters in much of their training. In palliative care the concern for meeting the needs of the whole person has prompted a greater understanding of spiritual issues, but there is little of what is done that can be classified as any more than awareness-raising. Despite this paucity, critical consideration has not been given to whether particular disciplines have any competence to sustain their claims for providing spiritual care and what the limits to this claim might be.

In an article on spiritual pain, Elsdon sets out what is a representative case for nurses to provide spiritual care for people who are terminally ill, a role in this case subsumed in the practice of nursing. In summary the argument is that, '[E]veryone experiences spiritual needs, whether or not they are part of a formal religious organisation, while only some have religious needs' (Elsdon 1995: 641). Comprehensive needs assessment is vital for the delivery of effective care, and if spiritual needs are accurately assessed and followed by appropriate interventions then it is possible to prevent spiritual distress. 'Nurses spend more time with terminally ill patients than most; they are often the ones to whom a patient will turn in spiritual distress, and are therefore in an excellent position to assess and help a person with spiritual pain' (ibid.: 642). Spiritual care is provided by the nurse in listening and giving attention to the patient, referring the patient to a chaplain or appropriate minister, praying with the patient, reading inspirational texts, reminiscing and providing music.

This general approach to spiritual care relies upon an understanding of the proposition of holistic care, an ability to identify conflicts in the patient's beliefs and to recognize the spiritual origin of pain, and 'being with' patients for this purpose. Heyes-Moore (1996) refers to no specific discipline in suggesting that:

> Effective help implies that the carer is fully present in relationship to the sufferer, person to person, deep calling to deep. The process of helping is based on the ill person finding meaning, through this dialogue, in his or her life experiences. Words, touch, symbolic imagery and rituals may all be vehicles for this unfolding story, which is, in essence, a contemplative process. It may truly be said that a person is healed by this in becoming whole while at the same time dying, so that death itself is not seen as a disaster but part of life.
>
> (Heyes-Moore 1996: 313)

The tenet of these examples appears reasonable, but there is little demonstrated in what is written that could be ascribed as professional practice in the strict sense that has been outlined above. Several ambiguities are present: the basis upon which spiritual care is being offered; the desirable end to which spiritual care is offered (other than relief of spiritual pain which is presumably a means to an end); the competence and constraints of the practitioner; the nature of the relationship between carer and patient; and the grounds for legitimizing the action taken. The desire to help perceived need in patients is an honourable compassionate response, but does it need to be more than this, and does it carry a greater moral responsibility than more generalized care? If spirituality is a fundamental dimension of being human then it surely merits not only care and attention but also the practice of sufficient competence, accountability, fidelity and discretion to merit the trust of those who turn to us for help.

A parallel set of issues to spiritual care can be seen in counselling, a term applied to a range of theories and practices that aim to help people cope with their existential and emotional problems. In palliative care, patients can be offered the opportunity to see a counsellor in order to work through issues which have arisen as a result of being diagnosed with a terminal disease and to help alleviate symptoms such as anxiety and depression. But counselling skills may be practised by any health professional, who may even use the title counsellor. Counselling theories and models have been absorbed by many 'helping' professionals and volunteers, and communication skills and counselling techniques are evident on medical syllabuses and specialist palliative medicine courses. The distinction between the two is not the intention but the grounds for rendering the practice of counselling based upon accredited training, continuing professional development and supervision, a public and professional accountability, a commitment to ethical practice and the interests of the patient. It is these duties and responsibilities which merit the trust of the patient to work with the counsellor and which provide the moral safeguards and protection of vulnerable people and their interests.

A professional ethic holds practitioners accountable for their acts and omissions, which is an important condition in obtaining trustworthiness. Accountability precedes as well as follows professional practice; it therefore encompasses at one end minimum codes of professional conduct outlining what can be expected, and at the other, procedures for addressing negligent practice and breaches of trust. The internal and external accountability of a profession maintains the reputation of competent practitioners, encourages their formation and reassures patients. This requires some means of regulating who should be admitted to the profession as well as a process of being able to remove and exclude those whose actions constitute unacceptable professional conduct or incompetence. The most visible form of accountability is the public register of members which generally sanctions the right to use the professional title, but registration is not uniform across the professions and it can denote a range of acceptable criteria. In counselling, regulation is provided through membership of professional bodies, but in spiritual care the only public registration is that provided by the faith communities of their licensed ministers, something which is by no means standard.

The issue of professional practice in spiritual care discloses wider debates in health care concerning the nature of orthodox practice, the grounds for therapeutic interventions and the moral nature of care. Educational and professional standards, competence and accountability are all part of these debates, perhaps most evident in the growing activity of complementary and alternative therapies. Most of these can be practised without any training, registration or regulation even though there are many emerging bodies seeking to demonstrate public responsibility (Mills and Peacock 1997). At the other end of the scale are the historic professions who wish to promote their own interests and safeguard not only the safety of patients but also their own standing and indispensability. There is good reason to suppose that the practice of spiritual care will not be disregarded in this respect and there seems good ethical justification that it should not continue without better accountability.

Standards of care

If spiritual care is to be practised with diligence and consistency then there must be some agreement about what this means in practice and how it can be achieved. It is simply an empty gesture to state in a service philosophy that the spiritual dimension is an important aspect of patient care, without embodying this in meaningful actions and useful resources. People are generally grateful for whatever care they receive and there are few expectations made of a service in terms of spiritual care, with the exception perhaps of seeing a chaplain at some time. But palliative care has rarely settled for the minimum in its active exploration of the needs of the whole person and the possibilities of care that it offers in response. Spiritual care should not be left shrouded in mystery, nor should it be hampered through uncertainty, but it should be actively engaged with and explored, as with any other aspect of care. If spiritual care is not robust enough to withstand this attention then it is probably best left as an obscure practice.

There are evident problems in trying to capture aspects of care in simplified forms, but in constructing models people are given the opportunity to share ideas and to debate and develop possibilities. This is part of the process that should be happening with spiritual care but of which there are few signs of activity. The prevalence of a generic spirituality in palliative care mitigates against a lead discipline which is further confounded by its limited cachet and low priority. However, spiritual care has not escaped the gaze of discriminating eyes entirely and it may be brought into an assessment of the overall quality of care provided by a service when it includes a comprehensive evaluation of how well the needs of patients are met (Glickman 1997).

The language of standards when used for evaluative purposes provides a benchmark against which to measure quality. Standards are a means of presenting a basic statement of what is required to achieve a desired practice. As an elementary description, standards are not comprehensive, but in their synopsis they provide an account of key factors deemed necessary in the provision of the particular aspect of care. We have already considered a critique of managed organizations in relation to spiritual care (Chapter 5) and noted the dangers of standardization and simplification. Standards as predetermined objectives bear the marks of their industrial genesis as performance indicators. Maxwell therefore cautions that:

> the last thing we need is the creation of some new Frankenstein's monster in the shape of a quality assurance or quality control scheme that is insensitive to the variation, autonomy, and trust implicit in health care. But it should not be beyond human wit to keep it simple, while providing a framework within which the quality of care may be studied, discussed, protected, and improved.
>
> (Maxwell 1984: 1471)

Few would disagree that spiritual care should be done well, but what it means to render good spiritual care requires the notion of quality to be considered in greater resolution. A statement in a service philosophy does not mean that spiritual care will happen; but, equally from what we have discussed, spirituality is not easily susceptible to a routine or predetermined course of action. However, that does not mean that we cannot outline some of the boundaries and suggest some of the contents. Spiritual care cannot just happen, there must be the purposeful application of certain resources, some level of ability to deal with spiritual issues within the care team, the appropriate use of skills and so forth. In addition, the quality of care may also include broader considerations such as its accessibility, equity, financial efficiency, benefits and the ethics of its practice.

Care standards are usually written in order that a service can be evaluated against them, good practice promoted and areas for development identified. This intention to audit necessarily suggests that standards must express elements of care that can be ascertained. Spiritual care depends upon practicalities as with many other aspects of care, and it should be able to be described at this level, given Maxwell's caution. As with all attempts to audit care there are questions of validity and reliability that need addressing as well as the practicality and ethics of the assessment process. Standards, by their very nature, are simplistic: they cannot allow for the subtleties and inevitable variance of interpersonal care, but they do provide a general indication of some elements of a service that should be expected, and no more than this. By auditing aspects of a service and comparing them to what are considered minimum or optimum standards, an estimation of quality can be gained, anecdote and intuition can be tested and some account of the service can be acquired.

Spiritual aspects of palliative care generally do not attract standards, something which can be regarded as a mixed blessing. But the absence of standards for spiritual care does little to integrate this dimension of palliative care into the overall quality of a service or further the development of good approaches to spiritual care. The obverse is that this absence may sustain inequities, problems with accessibility, poor practice and unmet needs. It may be that those involved in spiritual care feel that they lack the experience or expertise to write standards, but many services have multiprofessional audit groups who

Figure 6.1 Standard of spiritual care

Statement
The spirituality of patients and carers is acknowledged by the team, integrated within the care and support provided, and resources made available.

Structure
1 A spiritual care specialist (usually a chaplain) is readily available to provide and facilitate spiritual care for patients and carers.
2 The team has systems of communication with persons and bodies connected with different faiths who may be required for spiritual support.
3 Individuals have access to privacy and quiet, a room suitable for prayer, reflection and a place for religious observance (usually a chapel).
4 There is a suitable place for the patient to be visited after death.
5 There is provision within the patient documentation to record spiritual needs.

Process
1 Part of the initial multidisciplinary team assessment includes assessment of the spiritual health and care needs of the patient.
2 The team incorporates spiritual care into the patient's care plan in accordance with the wishes of the patient, or the patient's advocate.
3 There is a multidisciplinary review of the progress of spiritual issues and care needs.

Outcome
1 Patients, and their carers, state that they are aware of the people and facilities available to them to meet their spiritual care needs.
2 The patient and their carers indicate that they have been enabled to make progress with their spiritual concerns.

Source: Catterall *et al*. 1998: 166

should be able to assist and could even welcome the challenge. As with all attempts to write standards, it is vital to obtain the support and commitment of those who are involved in spiritual care. Glickman therefore advises that:

> The most successful approach to standard-setting is likely to involve a combination of consideration of published guidance from national bodies, learning from the practical experience of other units and services, and in-depth consultation within the organisation and with other interested parties.
>
> (Glickman 1997: 22)

An example of a standard of spiritual care is given in Figure 6.1. Like the Trent Hospice Audit Group's *Palliative Care Core Standards* (see Ahmedzai *et al.* 1998), this example uses the Donabedian model of quality: structure, process and outcome (Kogan and Redfern 1995). The standards published by the Trent Hospice Audit Group aim to be comprehensive and to 'dissect out what is commonly referred to as the "hospice philosophy"' (Ahmedzai *et al.* 1998: 18). The standard in Figure 6.1 was written in response and in addition to the seven published core standards of Ahmedzai *et al.* which included those of personal and cultural needs, psychosocial support and bereavement care and support. The standard in Figure 6.1 aims to realize an integrated philosophy of care in an integrated model of practice. The systems approach of the Donabedian model supports the interrelated aspects of care. In this case it is expressed in the involvement of the multidisciplinary team, the integration of the spiritual dimension into the care process, and the provision of systems, personnel and resources to facilitate spiritual care. Finally, the awareness of patients and carers of the provision of spiritual care and their progress with spiritual concerns are the indicators that there has been a benefit to patients.

Standards are not just assertions of good care but are intended to be verifiable. This dictates what can be contained in standards and angles them towards the obvious facets of care. Good care involves more than this in whatever field is considered and there is the danger that what is not measured is discounted in its value. Aspects of spiritual care deal with metaphors, narrative, ritual, transcendence, the sublime and the sacred, much of which is destroyed when it is forced to yield to a simplistic metric.

It is the organized, consistent, purposeful, resourced approach to spiritual care that paves the way for the creative and diverse engagement with the intangible and elusive. Palliative care services need to be encouraged to draft standards of spiritual care but they need equally to remember the caveats, for in more general terms, 'The arm around the shoulder, the ubiquitous cup of tea in time of crises, the person who does not know what to do or say but is kind and stays with you anyway – these are gestures that are both useless and powerfully caring' (Pattison 1996: 32).

Knowledge, skills and training

One of the reasons that people are prepared to approach palliative care services and put their trust in strangers is because staff are competent to deal with their needs. It is expected by patients that both within the team, and in particular people, there will be a body of specialist knowledge and skills that will be helpful and beneficial. In addition, staff are presumed to be properly trained to undertake their duties and to be accountable for their actions or inactions. When we consider the issues of spiritual care we have frequently observed that in general this is not an area that is addressed adequately or consistently in training, and this view is reinforced in the report *Education in Palliative Care* which states that:

> Like much else central to palliative care, these issues are seldom dealt with in post-graduate/post-qualifying education except in theological courses and in special courses run for or by specialists in palliative care . . .

(NCHSPCS 1996: 13)

Reasons for this deficiency can readily be found and generally focus upon the low priority afforded spiritual care within syllabi, the premise that there is an insubstantial knowledge and skills base for spiritual care, and that it is difficult to find recognized expertise. These are embedded within the wider debates about the philosophy of palliative care, the emphases given to the different perspectives on illness, the approaches to care which are validated and the roles and competences of team members. Training that addresses spiritual issues in palliative care is typically piecemeal, often synonymous with issues concerning culture, different faiths and customs around death, and seldom integrated into professional development. Different disciplines place different emphases upon the dimension and its inclusion or omission in core and specialist training. These differentials are exacerbated by the dearth of a consistent and developed approach to spirituality in national frameworks and guidelines.

The homogeneous spirituality favoured by palliative care obscures the underlying details and the plurality of discourses which engage with its many facets. Most notable are the faith communities which have highly developed doctrines, philosophies and teaching traditions. There are also academic schools such as philosophy, theology, psychology and sociology which address the phenomena and experiences of spirituality. All these approaches have generated their own libraries of knowledge, forms of analysis, schemes of description and accounts of spirituality. These various reflections contribute to a rich understanding of spirituality in its diverse expressions and experience and provide a fertile ground for study and a counterbalance to attempts at homogenizing this manifold feature of human life and history.

It can be expected that chaplains should have studied at least the spirituality of the faith tradition which they represent and have experience and a developed awareness of how a belief system personally operates. This would be an unreasonable expectation for any other discipline although it may of course be coincidental. Perhaps what is needed are not spiritual polymaths but the development of an active dialogue between the disciplines of palliative care and the disciplines that engage with spirituality focused on the themes of suffering, life-threatening illness and death. This may go some way in correcting a myopia of reductionism and to introducing a richness of perspectives. It will inevitably expose some of the cherished philosophy

Figure 6.2 A framework of care

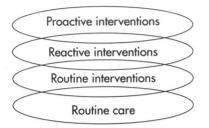

and practice of palliative care to scrutiny from outside its own tradition and introduce conflicting understandings. But this is surely preferable to a limited vocabulary that is comfortably familiar and yet plainly insufficient.

Developing and broadening the knowledge base for spirituality in palliative care will inform approaches to spiritual care and provide alternative perspectives from which to consider practices. Moral philosophy is one such view which brings many important questions to spiritual care, some of which have been introduced in the course of this book. Through this critical interaction concepts are shaped and modified, assumptions are revised and practice evolves and changes through being exposed to different insights, understandings and meanings. What, for example, can we learn about the care of the dying from concepts of death developed outside of the western religions? Are attitudes to suffering influenced by how people understand the sacred in contemporary society? Does a spiritual plurality present any psychological problems? How does a secular approach to death influence those who have to live with loss?

This grand scheme for engaging the palliative care accounts and experiences of spirituality with wider discourses is a necessary development. At a more immediate level are the issues of training and education that have to address the practical needs of disciplines providing care. Here the life contexts and narratives of patients suggest their own questions and dilemmas which should be addressed in the clinical and conceptual knowledge that relates to spiritual care. There will be a range of knowledge and skills required which reflect levels of competence appropriate to need. We can consider, in Figure 6.2, a simple arbitrary framework of care to illustrate something of this range which, for convenience, is arranged vertically.

- Routine aspects of care designate the unobtrusive but essential modes of care that are manifest through interpersonal relationships, communication, physical and non-physical attention, awareness of another's worldview and the impact of environment upon a person. In terms of spiritual care this concerns a sensitivity to a person's spiritual orientation, ensuring that the various dimensions of someone's spirituality are supported and that matters of space and place are included. Spiritual care at this level should include all those who have patient involvement, and forms part of basic clinical skills and knowledge. This is a competence that seems reasonable to require of all staff and therefore should be a core aspect of practice.

- Routine interventions are the common activities that take place between a patient and a particular discipline and which intrude into the patient's life. This can include activities directed at a particular patient such as the observations and assessments made by nurses and doctors, and regular treatments and procedures. Spiritual care in relation to this would involve the discernment and active assessment of spiritual needs, the identification of issues arising from the patient's spiritual orientation that need addressing and regular input of spiritual care, which for example might be in the form of a number of sessions with the chaplain. At this level, sufficient skills and knowledge would enable a fuller exploration of a patient's spirituality and may equip professionals to respond to a range of needs. Competence at this level would probably be expected of a core clinical team.

- Reactive interventions are responses to problems, concerns or needs arising outside of routine assessments that have not been anticipated. The onset of pain, anxiety or other symptoms; an event or experience (not necessarily clinical) in a patient's life which has a significant impact, or the result of making a particular choice may present a situation that calls for reactive intervention. For example, a terminally ill patient who has not wished to explore his spirituality or expressed any explicit spiritual needs discloses that he believes his deceased mother visited him in the night and that he now knows everything is going to be all right. The patient states that he would like to talk to someone about what the experience means and about 'what happens when you die'. Spiritual care would involve enabling an exploration of this experience as well as the patient's beliefs and understanding of death. This may provide the patient with an opportunity to face issues of mortality and consider beliefs about postmortem survival. There may also be a desire for some ritual aspect of faith or a wish to discuss and plan the funeral. There will be few teams who have an expert in 'near death' experiences but such experiences are not rare (Cherry 1995) and the issues that they raise fall within the spiritual domain. The scope of competence in a care team may be restricted to supporting the patient and allowing him the opportunity to express his understanding of the experience. The situation may suggest a number of concerns that may require referrals to specific disciplines within or outside of the team.

- Proactive interventions follow from anticipated concerns or situations as a result of an assessment, a predicted outcome based upon present conditions, or new circumstances arising which will have a future impact. The expected loss of function, the onset of the terminal phase, or something determined a potential risk may be considered situations where proactive interventions are required. For example, at a weekly multidisciplinary meeting the social worker raises her concern for the young daughter whose mother is dying. The daughter believes that her mother will go to heaven where 'she will be able to look down upon me'. The mother has told her daughter that heaven does not exist and when she dies she will know nothing of her daughter. These conflicting beliefs are already causing difficulties between the mother and daughter, and the social worker anticipates that it may present a particular issue in the grief and mourning of the child. This scenario suggests a need to understand something of the way that beliefs operate and develop in children, the child's understanding of dying and death and the significance of postmortem destiny in facing loss. Professional carers may have developed considerable experience in working with children, or there may be colleagues to whom they can refer. It may be necessary to involve a professional who has an understanding of the faith development of children and who can provide expertise. This is an example of a high level of skills and knowledge that requires a range of competences to be performed with considerable ability.

The level of different knowledge and skills suggested by these scenarios provides some indication of the range of abilities and training required. Spiritual care, as with many other aspects of care, requires general and specific competences and it cannot be expected that people will naturally possess such ability because spirituality is a human trait. A parallel can be drawn here from the approach to the care of bereavement found in palliative care. Bereavement is recognized as a common human experience: we all have some experience at some level of loss, most have indirect and many have direct experiences of bereavement. But this is not considered sufficient of itself to provide care for the bereaved. Firstly, there is the issue of carers projecting their own grief onto those who are seeking support. Secondly, being with bereaved people can be emotionally demanding and painful, which some carers are unable to sustain. Thirdly, while carers may be compassionate and empathetic, they work at different levels, have acquired different skills and abilities and will have different limits.

In spiritual care, professionals face similar issues, but these can be overlooked in the expectation that spiritual care can be provided somehow by everyone. This approach discourages the validity of limits and the development of particular skills and expertise. The cultivation of training is equally unlikely to occur if spiritual care is represented as a benign and inevitable aspect of palliative care dissociated from the external discourses of spirituality. A final but important parallel with training in bereavement care is the time typically given for self-reflection and attending to personal experiences of loss so that a level of self-awareness is developed. The 'private' character of a person's spiritual orientation is often used as a defence to avoid addressing this aspect in training, but while spirituality is certainly personal it is inevitably expressed in a person's values and beliefs which guide their actions, attitudes and the meaning of experiences, both their own and those of the people they care for.

The provision of spiritual care is a matter not simply of adequate education but also of adequate practice and of professional formation. Knowledge guides practice and may dictate technical proficiency but the spiritual dimension of palliative care is more than a process of applying abstract knowledge, principles and theory. The assumption is doubtful that if anything is to be credible and valid it must be captured in systematic knowledge provided through scientific techniques. There is an 'increasing acceptance that important aspects of professional competence cannot be represented in propositional form and be embedded in a publicly accessible knowledge base' (Eraut 1994: 15). This is therefore a question not just of the relationship of theory to practice but of how we should train carers, for no matter how extensive a curriculum is it will never be adequate to the irrational, intangible and manifold spiritual dimension. Schön (1987) poses the dilemma by means of a graphic analogy:

> In the varied topography of professional practice, there is a high hard ground overlooking a swamp. On the high ground, manageable problems lend themselves to solution through the application of research-based theory and technique. In the swampy lowland, messy, confusing problems defy technical solution. The irony of this situation is that the problems of the high ground tend to be relatively unimportant to individuals or society at large, however great their technical interest may be, while in the swamp lie the problems of greatest human concern. The practitioner must choose. Shall he remain on the high ground where he can solve relatively unimportant problems according to prevailing standards of rigor, or shall he descend to the swamp of important problems and nonrigorous inquiry?
>
> (Schön 1987: 3)

Patients do not generally present their spiritual orientations and needs in delineated ways that conform to textbook cases for they are not systematic and their spirituality comes attached to the whole of their lives. The theory-based approach to care attempts to exclude or control the perplexity by applying a filter in order to identify an existing solution. But in using a necessarily narrow frame of reference, what is significant and important to a patient may go unnoticed. Pain provides an example of this, for it can be subjected to a number of existing physiological theories which indicate a pharmacological response, but pain means much more than this to the patient. 'Pain is the sign for something not answered; it refers to something open, something that goes on the next moment to demand what is wrong? How much longer? . . . Why does this kind of evil exist, and why does it strike just me?' (Illich 1976: 149). By applying a single frame we do not restrict the experience and meaning of pain to the patient but we block these off from the view of the carer and make pain the object of a technical skill and a rational problem. Spirituality viewed through a filter may become a problem of providing a particular diet or antidepressants, but, to use the above analogy, this will involve the professional moving away from the patient and stepping onto the highground.

Schön (1987) argues that because professionals have to deal with messy reality they need more than the teaching of academically rigorous knowledge and its application. Professionals need educating in the 'art' of clinical practice which concerns the abilities of perception, intuition, judgement and improvization which enable the practitioner to deal with the uniqueness of each individual they encounter. This is the basis for Schön's concept of 'reflective practice' which he explains as the capacity to develop intelligent actions by learning through what we do. In this way, routine responses from the standard repertoire become subject to a process in which they are shaped and developed in each situation in which they are being used. This does not bypass the need for professional knowledge and facts, or the ability to apply them, but from this professionals can learn to deal with uncertain contexts of patients' lives. If we apply this to the spiritual aspects of palliative care we can see how professionals may develop from a knowledge of spirituality to an 'art' of practice which in the end cannot be taught but must be learned.

The palliative care disciplines which include some form of spiritual care in their training curricula are generally based upon the cognitive goals of acquiring certain knowledge and understanding how this applies to patients. Curricula may also include discussion about appropriate 'skills' but it is in clinical practice, through supervision, mentoring and critical reflection that experiential learning takes place. In the USA there is the provision of clinical pastoral education which provides training in pastoral ministry based upon psychoanalytical and Judeo-Christian tradition which incorporates an established programme of hospital clinical placements. In Britain there is no such scheme although placements are established between theological colleges and hospitals, hospices and palliative care services. There are generally no structured opportunities for disciplines other than chaplains to develop spiritual care practices while this learning is presumed to take place within the professional training that disciplines undertake. There is little evidence that this is provided, and Oldnall's (1996) critical analysis of nursing may easily apply to other disciplines: 'For the most part, holistic care is defined as consisting solely of the biopsychosocial aspects of humanity, and appears to give little or no recognition to the impact and relevance of spirituality on the individual' (Oldnall 1996: 143). The inconsistencies between theory, practice and expectation of spiritual care do not cultivate a purposeful attitude to spiritual care, even less encourage the development of competent practice. Professional bodies who claim it is part of their discipline's role have not generally devoted much attention to how this may be learnt beyond the classroom, the levels of knowledge and ability that are required or the limits of practice.

In contrast to the national bodies, local palliative care services may provide educational opportunities in spirituality and spiritual care as part of their in-house training and their educational work. These may span a number of different levels, involve different disciplines and provide forums for reflecting upon experience. Case conferences and multidisciplinary team meetings may also be places in which reflection upon practice can take place and where less experienced professionals can observe the deliberative processes of more established colleagues and test their own understanding and knowledge. It is perhaps at this local level that some of the most creative dialogues and developments are taking place in this field but which rarely surface for wider dissemination. This may be inevitable given the comparatively undeveloped discourse of this domain, but it is regrettable that this silence is so often interpreted as an absence.

In considering a professional approach to the spiritual dimension of palliative care we return, however, to the contentious issues of what is proper spiritual care and who should be practising it, what qualifies them to do so, what standards should they be working to, what competences should be expected of them and what is the ethical framework of their practice. These are matters not only for disciplines that operate within palliative care but also for the claims of moral legitimacy and expertise by which professions merit the trust of society and negotiate the balance of interests between those of the patient, their own interests and the interests of society. In this respect the spiritual dimension of palliative care comes within the growing debate about the relevance and rigour of practices employed in the care of people with life-threatening conditions. However, perhaps the significant question in all this remains the one which is the least given to resolution: how should palliative care respond to what is an unavoidable aspect or reality for many people and that lifts human existence beyond the rational and mundane to endow life with profound meaning, not least in the face of death?

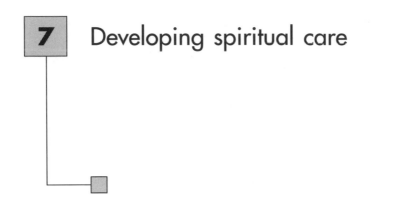

7   Developing spiritual care

Spirituality has been the focus of this book but it has by no means been its exclusive subject for as we have critically pursued the spiritual dimension of palliative care we have had to deal with a broad range of issues. Rather than treating spirituality in isolation we have firmly located it within overlapping and multilayered contexts and considered it from a number of perspectives. In this final chapter we revisit the major themes that have emerged in the course of our enquiries with the intention of outlining some of the major issues which may determine the future developments of spiritual care.

Spiritual pluralism

The fact that spirituality is to be found in the most basic definitions of palliative care is remarkable given the purportedly hostile environment of contemporary society and the inevitable materialism of an organized health service. The presence of spirituality in the accounts of palliative care bears witness not only to the historical legacy of hospice care but also to an enduring conviction and experience that human existence is more than a matter of flesh and blood. What the 'more' is has occupied the great minds of history, and in our day it is a question for science as much as it remains one of philosophy. Spirituality, however, attracts some condemnation including that of being a chimera – a mere illusion thrown up by our psyche to make life more bearable; a deceit – no more than a useful trick of consciousness and a product of evolution; and a myth – a primitive way of understanding the world that is untestable but scientifically false. There are any number of apologias for spirituality that can be rehearsed in its defence, but whatever position is taken, that people experience and express what they consider to be spiritual in their lives is unavoidable.

Palliative care as a multidisciplinary speciality recognizes the fact of the spiritual but more than this it cannot presume or question, for it does not lie within its scope. By recognizing the spiritual, palliative care allows for it in its philosophy, attends to it in those it cares for and may properly concern itself in studying spirituality in its relation to terminal illness, dying and death. Palliative care as a discipline can be no other than agnostic. Its concern is not in the proof of spirituality, only its presence manifest among those it strives to help. This means that the spirituality represented in palliative care aims to be generic and appeal to the broadest possible interpretation despite its own heritage. But spirituality gains its relevance and reason in its specific orientation, and therefore the unifying holistic theory regularly used in palliative care can be more problematic than helpful because it can fail to distinguish the importance and meaning of particular orientations. A spiritual plurality would be a far more realistic position for palliative care to adopt and is a better reflection of the reality which it faces. It is possible to consider that pluralism is also to some extent a characteristic of palliative care in general, most notable in the multidisciplinary approach that suggests a diversity of perspectives on illness. This provides space for the spiritual dimension in palliative care but it also subjects it to criticism both from those in faith traditions who censure spiritual pluralism for its disorientation and from those in biomedical traditions who find little account of the spiritual in the objectification of illness.

The spiritual dimension of palliative care requires an understanding that has less to do with utility and more to do with attending to another human being. This is a hermeneutic that encompasses the enigmatic nature of personhood that is encountered in suffering, dying and death. We can barely understand ourselves, less still another person, and yet we can draw close to another but know of the remoteness in the encounter. This paradox means that we cannot presume to articulate anything more than an intimation when we seek to describe the spiritual – hence the unspoken but present 'other' between two people. This brings us to the question of what language we can use to describe the spiritual whose syntax we struggle to grasp and for which we have only a vocabulary of approximation. It seems that metaphors, myths, symbols, ritual, art and music express something of the spiritual because through their transparency we recognize meaning beyond empirical fact. Therefore it may be the disciplines and therapists in palliative care who make use of these forms who are most able to articulate the spiritual and to encounter it in others. This language stands in relief to that which seeks to objectify and measure the human condition, but as a hesitant language it is rarely the first language to be spoken or heard.

Palliative care is, in its origins, a non-conformist movement, a protesting reaction to the postwar medical orthodoxy and an ideal that is imbued with a spiritual vision of humanity with faith in an ultimate destiny. This hope was beyond the grasp of medicine and it was one that helped to motivate the widespread development of this appealing form of the care of the dying and the revival of a modern *ars moriendi*. Part of the success of palliative care has also depended upon advances in medicine and the appropriation of its undeniably successful techniques and procedures. That the two can co-exist in palliative care is not surprising given the pluralistic perspectives that contribute to the care of the whole person. However, as palliative care returns increasingly to areas of health care where biomedicine is the dominant and privileged view, it remains to be seen if the spiritual dimension will be suppressed. However, medicine, as a profession and practice, has not been without challenge, discontent and problems. A more confident 'consumer' has registered dissatisfaction and exercised choice to the extent that a new medical pluralism may be emerging (Cant and Sharma 1999). It is in this pluralism that the return of palliative care to the place from which it departed may welcome the spiritual dimension in its manifest forms.

The presence of religion

Religion is a confounding phenomenon in contemporary society and an awkward subject for palliative care despite the religious roots of the care of the dying. Palliative care services are not religious communities but they maintain religious references and reflect something of the contemporary 'religious' life. This is another of the contexts in which the spiritual is located, and it is far more subtle, dynamic and resilient than the prophets of religion's demise had made allowances for. The multifaceted dimensions and spectrum of religious beliefs and practices subvert the simple yes or no account provided for in the perfunctory admission of patients. In addition, the common religion in Britain of Christian nominalism is a difficult form of religion to identify clearly, for which the succinct epithet of 'believing without belonging' provides a useful grasp but only a hint of the diversity it contains.

Traditional religion for many people no longer provides a substantial framework of beliefs and values, although it may inform some part of their world-view. This is why secularist assumptions can be problematic, because whilst the dynamics of modernity have displaced many of the social functions of religion it does not discount other dimensions, and in particular the sacred and spiritual dimensions. The absence of religion in the secularism of palliative care may enable it to express a proper openness to all people, but it may work against care of the whole person because it fragments religion as an aspect of patient life and frequently partitions it from the concept of spirituality. Some psychological theories assert that a dormant religion is revived at a time of crisis, although some research contradicts this thesis. But whatever the motivation for religious orientation, people may be supported and helped by their religious beliefs and practices which therefore may contribute to quality of life.

The presence of different faiths among the populations that are served by palliative care services introduces a series of challenges not the least of which are those about equity and accessibility. The different faith traditions also bring challenges to the practice of palliative care and to the concept of a homogeneous all-encompassing spirituality. Death, illness and suffering are universal experiences but they are understood within world-views that frame particular meanings. Services can usually accommodate the more objective elements of different religions but meanings, values and beliefs require more than alternative facilities and resources. The differences in approach among primary, secondary and tertiary care settings may present possibilities for dialogue in order to develop an understanding of palliative care in relation to different faiths. It may also throw into relief the implicit world-views of a service, the service providers and the meanings which people assume.

The secularization theories suggest that these frames are crumbling fast and that people are no longer embedded within cohesive belief systems or rooted within tradition. The established religions are deemed incompatible with contemporary life in which their plausibility is challenged by other authorities and their world-view is one among many to choose from. But the dissolution of religion has not happened in the way suggested by the postulated secular society. Religion persists but takes on different forms, and one that finds particular correspondence in palliative care is that of the New Age. The self-spirituality of the New Age can be considered as a contemporary religious expression that is utopian, holistic and which recognizes a universal spirituality of humanity. The primacy of self-experience and expression contrasts with received beliefs of traditional religious orthodoxy, relocating the sacred and providing an alternative source of authority. The hospice and New Age movements have arisen within the same social milieu and both challenge and reinterpret tradition. Perhaps both also complement the individual search for meaning and for (inner) healing in the face of death.

If modernity questions religion's plausibility, it also challenges the tenability of orthodox medical practice – with both being subject to doubt, a diminution of authority and a growing willingness of individuals to seek alternatives. The formation of hospice and palliative care can be located within this cultural shift in which there is still a trace of religion but only a hint of any theology. Religion has become detached from a vocation to care and has been renamed a special need and a matter for the individual. But whilst this represents a credible position for a public service it squanders the religious explorations of illness, suffering and death. It is surely a matter of regret that the presence of religion in palliative care is limited to patient need and that through pursuing expediency a significant feature of human life and history is neglected.

Exploring death

It may be thought that death is the focus of palliative care, but death is also its termination. Dying and the management of the terminally ill is the central concern of palliative care, and whilst it can do much to redeem the concluding days of life it will never be able to allay death itself. But how death is understood and what it means to die will affect not only the way the terminally ill approach their death but also the way the living attend to the dying (Neuberger 1999). This is why palliative care must attend to the meanings of death both for patients and for those who provide care. What does the end of life mean for a particular person with a fatal illness, for those who are directly involved with that person and for the wider community in which that person lives and dies? Not only does palliative care intercept these meanings but it also enacts its own meanings that impact upon the experience and understanding of death. In particular, through a disproportionate and popular presence in the public arena, hospice care is symbolic of an understanding of the end of life which is particularly evident in moral and legal debates about the manner and timing of death.

To the question, 'What is death?', we can only attempt to provide one-sided answers, but although death is a boundary and border which contains the living this has not stopped us from considering what lies beyond. Here we encounter the religious, artistic and philosophical imaginations which seek to make sense of our mortal human condition and of the unknown in which lies our destiny. For some, death represents a horizon over which there is a continuation of the self; for others death represents a complete end to self save for that which persists in their legacy. Whatever is believed about death refers back to life and to what is considered to be fundamentally important and meaningful. Therefore death can be understood as a focus for the spiritual because it brings the living to reflect upon what they believe about the nature of personhood and the experiences of being in the world, of being in relationship with others and of the intangible, the numinous and the sacred.

Enabling people to explore the meaning of death is regarded as a proper concern of palliative care. But whilst this assertion is often stated it is seldom clarified. In practice the justified interest that prompts enquiries into bowel movements and intimate relationships seldom extends to someone's view of human destiny unless specifically initiated by the patient or their carers. The spiritual agnosticism of palliative care and the centrality of patient autonomy suggest that individuals are supported in finding, affirming or possibly reconstructing their own meaning. However, meanings are not self-generated; affirmation requires external validation and reconstruction suggests some idea of form or pattern. This apparent contradiction also seems to disregard other frames of meaning not least that which palliative care surrounds death in its convictions, implicit values and practices. Palliative care endows death with significance and meaning beyond the crude biological facts, although it may be difficult to deduce from this anything more than a vague spiritual direction. This can be regarded as a reflection of the spirit of the age or it might be considered a disservice to those struggling with anomie and disorientation. A solution, however, is offered in the provision of the 'expert' to whom patients can be referred for particular counsel, but whilst a patient with a discernible spiritual orientation may suggest who the relevant guide should be, there are those without a clear direction who may be more problematic in this respect. The problem, however, is removed if it is accepted that death is either a substantially private concern or without meaning.

If postwar medicine sequestrated death, and modern society has privatized the meaning of death, then palliative care has perhaps made a further move by developing a specialism around death, or more accurately the processes leading to death and their consequences. Death within a specialism supports the personal approach to death and helps to maintain a substantially extrinsic relationship to society, but it may also construct meaning through its growing sense of tradition and by framing the individual experience within a collective movement. To some extent this specialist meaning can be considered self-referential, but in the dispersion of palliative care into acute and community settings there will be an unavoidable encounter with other sources of meaning and different interpretations of death. A more pluralistic environment may have the benefit of both an attenuated professional discourse and a resonant context of habits, history and identity which provide their own narratives and practices. However, these social and cultural resources are vulnerable to the conformity and dislocation of institutionalized lay and professional roles even though they may be significant sources of eschatology and hope.

This myopic, but practical, view of death is further exemplified in the care provided to the bereaved where the focus is typically upon predefined grief pathology and the risks of psychosocial transition. Meanings and beliefs about death, which may be significant factors in grief, do not usually merit inclusion on assessment forms and are likely to be excluded from many schools of counselling. In the care of the living and the dying, palliative care can be understood as focused substantially upon and limited to the body which becomes its object. Clinical observations of patients through to the physical management of grief set the visible and embodied self over and above the more intangible aspects of personhood (Hallam *et al.* 1999). By contrast, discourses that are not confined to the physical body, such as the spiritual, may become subordinated even though they can encompass significant aspects of mortality and bereavement. It could be argued that all but the physical is beyond the reach of palliative care, but it is the argument of this book that the end of life demands a far more nuanced and expansive approach that challenges such differentiation and is responsive to the enriching narratives of death which shape our understanding and practice.

Spiritual care by whom?

The holistic philosophy popular in palliative care supplies two key justifications, used by different disciplines, to be involved with spiritual care: caring for the totality of the person means that the spiritual is unavoidable; and because we are all spiritual we all have the capacity to provide spiritual care. It is an argument that has little purchase with regards other aspects of care and is perhaps symptomatic of the conceptual ambiguity and the professional presumption in this field. Spirituality is the proper concern of all those who have a role in patient care, but it is difficult to accept how a concern can bear the weight of a professional duty or underpin a claim to expertise. Attending to human need requires compassion and the expectation of beneficence which should be the foundation of all care and none of which is proprietary. In order to facilitate spiritual care and to achieve a trustworthy service there needs to be more specific goals and obligations. These are enabled by knowledge, skills and a public commitment to duty that is prescribed by an orientation to a particular good. It is therefore in promoting the spiritual good of a patient, and not in expertise or contracts, that we can establish the grounds for a legitimate professional practice in spiritual care.

There is no franchise or licence to be had for spiritual care in Britain; the closest we have to authorized practitioners are the clergy whose denominations publicly affirm the vows of those called to the spiritual service of others. The modern hospice movement adopted the practice of hospitals in appointing clergy to be their chaplains to provide for the spiritual needs of patients and to some extent this has continued in palliative care. It is the client who extends trust to the professional, and it is the patient who may refuse or accept the offer of a chaplain to promote their spiritual good. A concern by a professional for a patient's spiritual welfare, if it has been expressed at all, cannot generate anything more than a vague expectation by a patient of what assistance may be offered. By contrast, the role of the clergy, in as much as it is in the public domain, represents a shared and specific set of expectations and responsibilities. It is on this basis that patients and their carers can choose to put their trust in a chaplain to provide help with their spiritual needs if they so wish.

An holistic philosophy provides a very weak justification for allowing any health professional *carte blanche* to undertake any aspect of promoting a patient's best interests. This would require either collapsing certain limits of professional discretion or the devaluation of all spiritual interests to some superficial notion of well-being. The professions claiming that they have a role in responding to spiritual need, therefore, should be clear what it is they are offering and on what basis. Patients may well disclose their spiritual concerns to anyone they choose, but this does not constitute an expectation that the chosen person will be able to respond. If a response is made, what is its motivation and the framework in which it takes place? There is often much confusion in the professional literature concerning these matters and a failure to explore them critically. It may be tedious to keep reworking the ground of definitions, concepts, theories and clinical models, but spiritual care is in danger of limited development if it does not tend to its foundations. Spiritual care also needs to form part of the wider dialogue in palliative care about the nature of supportive care and the relationship between the spiritual, social, psychological and physical aspects of living and dying.

The dichotomy between the general ideals of palliative care and the reality of practice should raise some serious questions about who delivers spiritual care. This is both the internal debate of a specialism as well as one which is located in a wider sociological and cultural context. It concerns the large philosophical questions of human existence and being as well as the immediate practical questions of who can be trusted to help those with the dilemmas raised by mortality. The place and role of religion, and particularly that of Christianity and its clergy, is a significant issue for this debate in the West. However, in a strangely similar way to the position of death in contemporary culture, religion is both absent and present. It also frequently bears the inscriptions of prejudice and is often sequestered to avoid serious engagement. This also presents a challenge to the many ministers of religion appointed as chaplains who are involved in palliative care teams to engage with their colleagues in other disciplines in exploring the nature of spiritual care through rigorous dialogue. There is also a challenge to theology to demonstrate that it is a practical discipline (Elford 1999) and one which can make a particular contribution to the discourses of palliative care.

The field seems to be left wide open at the moment for spiritual care to be claimed as a legitimate aspect of the professional practice of any number of disciplines. Ironically, the chaplain can be technically exempted from this domain by being classed as a religious specialist and therefore subject to segregation from those who profess no corresponding belief system. But assisting people in their spiritual search is too important a matter to be appended to the role of anyone who subscribes to an holistic approach of care. There needs to be a more discerning and thorough means of ensuring that not only are the people offering spiritual care equipped with necessary skills and sensitivity, but that they are morally obligated to the spiritual good of the patient. Most crucially, it is care which moves beyond the conventional approach dependent upon expertise and into an encounter between two vulnerable human beings alert to the creative possibilities of transcendence despite being grounded in life's fragility. It is, therefore, care formed out of the deepest human experience and directed towards profound human needs which exist despite good physical, social and psychological care. This is the professional challenge and the daunting task of anyone who claims to work in this field.

The directions of spiritual care

Spiritual care has undergone considerable movement since the birth of the modern hospice. Much of this movement has involved a distancing of spirituality from religion and more particularly from Christianity which was such a significant influence on the founding, most notably, of St Christopher's Hospice and on the work of Cicely Saunders (Clark 1998). The expansion and development of the hospice movement and the shifting social and cultural climate provided the momentum for change but there has been a discernible divergence in the direction this change has taken. On the one hand there has been the move towards a more existential and eclectic notion of spirituality, which is individually based and validated, as opposed to an externally validated and appropriated religious form of spirituality. On the other hand there has been the move towards an institutionally recognized and systematic form of spirituality that involves its objectification and management. Between these two there remains forms of Christian pastoral care and ritual practice prevalent at both an individual and an institutional level.

Developments in spiritual care have often been to the advantage of healthcare professionals who have either rediscovered or readily adopted a spiritual aspect in their practice. A subjective spirituality uncoupled from a systematic theology can become assimilated into the tolerant humanism that is manifest in many of the values operationalized by healthcare professionals. This detraditionalized spirituality presents a widespread therapeutic benefit and can be accommodated easily within an autonomy-based approach to care. Spiritual care may thus become another competence to be acquired by the practitioner striving to deliver holistic care and another process in an organization focused on outcomes. But this saves spirituality as a whole from sequestration and positions some form of it alongside other aspects of care to be considered. This enables the spiritual domain to be kept in view and to be some part of the palliative care discourse which consequently brings it within the framework of managed organizations.

The mobility of palliative care philosophy has also provided new directions for spiritual care outside of specialist units. In primary, secondary and tertiary sectors of health care there has been something of an awakening to the benefits of the palliative care approach. This presents considerable challenges for spiritual care, especially when it becomes less dependent on a hospice and more reliant upon peripatetic services. It also raises questions of where the responsibilities lie for spiritual care within communities and what it means to them. Common to all settings are concerns of quality, assessment of needs, effectiveness, accessibility, equity and cost. It also invites the inevitable comparison of spiritual care between different settings and brings into focus any disparities in resources. Such an exercise will shape a demanding agenda for spiritual care, not least for the sort of research required to provide a rigorous evidence base for future developments.

Spirituality in palliative care is often presented as a benign overarching or underpinning concept of humanity, but its existence as an homogeneous concept is impugned when it is considered in relationship to different faith traditions. The diverse cultures of humankind are diminished in attempting neat syntheses, and distinct spiritual orientations are disrespected if they are classed as essentially similar. However, within limits, we can find common ground and ways of approaching spiritual traditions that are sensitive to different experiences, practices and philosophies. Death and suffering are common to humanity but are looked upon in many ways by the world's religions, each of which may have important things to say about the care of the dying. However, this dialogue is disabled when a reductionist approach is taken to spirituality and professionals are unaware of the influence of their own spiritual orientation. It therefore requires some bold initiatives to move beyond the safety of a spiritual tourism that is often evident in educational programmes, and towards a deeper recognition and understanding of different spiritual views.

Spirituality viewed from outside of the established palliative care community does not just concern different spiritual traditions because it also takes us beyond the confines of cancer. Living and dying with a non-malignant disease may raise incomparable spiritual issues distinguished by the meaning of the illness as much as by its pathological progression. It seems reasonable to suggest, therefore, that there may be spiritual care needs characteristic of, say, progressive neurological disorders as contrasted with cancer. Where palliative care is extended towards a more generic form then it is probable that spiritual care will develop in new ways shaped by the experiences of those living and dying with terminal diseases other than cancer. Whilst it can be argued that this already happens in acute care and to some extent in community care, within palliative care the dominant paradigm for spiritual care is cancer. To what extent patients suffering with non-malignant fatal diseases are the 'disadvantaged dying' (George and Sykes 1997: 252) in terms of spiritual care has yet to be fully explored, but there is certainly a moral case to be made for some form of an equivalent service to be available.

A professional spiritual care?

There is a reticence within palliative care to attribute the professional adjective to the spiritual domain. The reticence is a symptom of the uncertainty with which people approach spiritual care as well as the defended power and influence of professional status. It also suggests that palliative care generally holds spirituality to be benign and therefore affords those who deal with it an unusually high level of trust. The idea of vocation rather than profession is typically invoked when talking about chaplains, although this is usually shorthand for the theological aspect of their motivation. However, this invocation is not an argument against chaplains as a profession but a means of distinguishing them from other professionals or delineating a religious from a secular vocation. None of this exempts those who care for the spiritual well-being of patients from the extraordinary commitment to beneficence and compassion that should be expected from those who attend them. Nor does it remove the moral obligation for competence in those who profess to practise spiritual care. But it does help to obstruct a usefully rigorous engagement with spirituality and its accompanying issues.

Developing a professional approach to spiritual care requires that conflicting interests are recognized and addressed. There should be an interdisciplinary approach among healthcare professionals, but there should also be dialogue among the academic faculties whose gaze includes spirituality. Spirituality in the context of palliative care is left relatively undisturbed by wider studies and debates and yet it has so much to gain by engaging with them. However, spirituality may also be left undisturbed within palliative care, where minimal expectations and uncertain practice may leave spiritual care low on standards and peripheral to the delivery of good care. Standards of spiritual care are not going to provide instant redress to these shortcomings, but they should encourage a more consistent, purposeful and resourced approach. Perhaps of equal value, the process of producing standards in this domain will encourage those involved in delivering palliative care to step onto the hallowed ground which has been considered until recently out of bounds to all but the few.

Knowledge, skills and training will provide important platforms in developing a professional approach to spiritual care. If chaplaincy is to be the lead discipline in this field then it must be conspicuous in contributing the specialist knowledge and skills it has developed. The healthcare professionals who practise spiritual care should seek to broaden their knowledge base as well as define more clearly the scope of their competence. A range of knowledge and skills needs to be matched by a range of training and education. There also needs to be some means of validating understanding and practice in order to demonstrate an ability to provide spiritual care. But this drift towards a conventional professional approach is not without its problems.

Spiritual care is grounded in being human, and it therefore draws as much upon the caring person as it does technique. Self-understanding, reflection and self-discipline are as necessary as the application of knowledge in the encounters that take place in spiritual care. Therefore a professional approach to spiritual care will recognize that therapeutic techniques are encompassed within a broader *art* of clinical practice that is acquired through a rigorous process of professional formation. Inevitably this way of training will be more apparent and realizable to certain disciplines.

Professionals act on behalf of and for the benefit of others. Healthcare professionals therefore develop relationships with patients which are distinctly different from the relationship that exists through contractual obligations or the social functions implied by a specified role. Campbell (1984) argues that the professional relationship is a form of detached love which balances reason and emotion in reaching out to another in need:

> what professional carers have to offer to society (in return for the undoubted advantages they receive from it) is the 'moderation of love'. This has been shown to be both a skill (the subtle balance between involvement and detachment) and a symbolic role (the mediation of concern and hope for the individual, even in the most dire illness and distress).
>
> (Campbell 1984: 126)

To state the obvious, professional carers have deeply human relationships with those they care for with all the potential and difficulty that accompany them. This is why healthcare professionals not only need to ground their relationships in a clear commitment to the good of the vulnerable patient but also to develop the ability to be involved in another's life within particular limits. A professional approach to spiritual care must equally demonstrate these characteristics and realize responsibilities that accompany a symbolic role. The roles of the doctor, nurse and chaplain are all symbolic of the human need for health and healing and human flourishing. In the context of palliative care, these meanings acquire a mortal perspective and the chaplain in particular becomes symbolic of human destiny and the transcendence of mortality. Symbolic roles which concern the mediation of important human goods typically exercise significant authority in society which can so easily distort relationships. If a profession is to practise spiritual care then it must do so with all the safeguards to trust that are needed to legitimize the authority which people are willing to invest in it.

Spiritual care is seldom treated to such a rigorous ethical enquiry and this is to the detriment of patients and to those who work in palliative care. This is not principally a matter of trying to place spiritual care onto some safe moral highground but of ensuring that there is rigorous and reasoned argument to justify what should or should not be considered good practice within palliative care. Not everything that takes place under the banner of palliative care needs to be carried out by professionals, but it seems reasonable to consider that the spiritual dimension of humanity is a sufficient weighty matter in the face of death to require considerable care and the utmost caution.

Conclusion

> Like as the waves make towards the pebbled shore,
> So do our minutes hasten to their end;
> Each changing place with that which goes before,
> In sequent toil all forwards do contend.
>
> (Sonnet 60, Shakespeare)

In facing the inevitability of death we face both what is certain and what is unfamiliar, what is plain fact and what is incomprehensible. The enigma of death is approached by a number of health-related disciplines with their own techniques and frames of reference, but there remains vast territories outside of this region with which humanity contends. If palliative care seeks to support people in facing death beyond the material reality then it needs to recognize and respond to the spiritual experiences and intimations that point towards profound aspects of human nature and destiny. An awareness of human finitude prompts many people to reflect upon this wider view that is not limited to accounts of the immediate facts:

> Imagine you're dangling above a ravine at the end of a weak rope. In that situation you will listen breathlessly to the instructions of a man who knows how much the rope can withstand before it snaps. But following such an experience you would not call this rope expert a life expert, someone who knows all about the human condition. For that something else is needed.
>
> (Keizer 1997: 169)

What is needed for spiritual care has been the subject of the second part of this book in which we have explored some of the theory and practice that relates to this aspect of palliative care. It should by now be apparent that this is a field which is replete with assumptions but short on creative dialogue and critique. Spirituality in palliative care may for some people be too peripheral to warrant serious consideration, for others it may represent too dangerous a place to venture both personally and professionally. But palliative care does not exist in a social vacuum and it seems incongruous within this wider context that there is an apparent contentment to continue promoting an ideology of spiritual care without engaging at least with the culture in which it is located (Clark and Seymour 1999: 179).

In this concluding section we shall draw upon the arguments presented in the course of this book to suggest some of the areas that need addressing. This is not an attempt to outline a comprehensive agenda for change because there is too much preliminary work that needs to be undertaken before that position is reached. Nor is it an attempt to distil neat solutions from a complex mixture of themes and factors. But what we can undertake is the siting of a few signposts that may prove useful in providing some direction to the development of spiritual care. Signposts are not always found as useful as those who set them up anticipate, and consequently they may not be as permanent as was first expected. The following three signposts invite the ramblers and explorers in palliative care not only to try out the directions they point towards but also to feed back whether or not they need relocating or repositioning.

Research

It has been reiterated in many of the preceding discussions that there is a paucity of research concerning spirituality in palliative care. Research is not a prominent activity within palliative care as a whole compared with other areas of health care. There is a proper sensitivity and ethical constraint in subjecting people to research, particularly towards the end of life. But as palliative care becomes more established earlier on in the disease trajectory and in life-enhancing care such as rehabilitation, then research is likely to become more practicable and justified. Research in the field of spirituality is beset with the obvious problem of how to investigate aspects of what is intangible or immaterial. However, spirituality is not alone in this problem and it has some very tangible effects that can be observed and studied through relevant or correlated variables such as people's behaviour, beliefs and clinical outcome (Holland *et al.* 1999; King *et al.* 1999). Spirituality is not a discrete unidimensional concept and its close interrelation to other variables requires a clear explanation of what can be inferred from observation.

Quantitative and qualitative approaches both have their place in researching spirituality in palliative care. Whether we are considering spiritual care as an aspect of service delivery or the effect of spirituality upon patients' quality of life, there is likely to be relevant experience in other fields that can be drawn upon. If research in this domain is to be credible it will need to be systematic and rigorous in order to maximize the accuracy of the results and to minimize confounding factors and bias. The design of the study, the method of data collection, the type of analysis undertaken and the means of interpretation will probably have to withstand the scrutiny of ethics committees and may also be subject to the examination of funding bodies. But any research undertaken should be able to demonstrate a necessary rigour to justify the investment of resources, the intrusion into the lives of patients, and the implications of results (Bowling 1997).

Research will be crucial in developing some form of an evidence base for spiritual care. This presents palliative care with the opportunity for collaboration among disciplines, to question the ample anecdotes in this field and to investigate assumptions. The case of need for spiritual care is one example that seems an obvious candidate for researchers, but it raises many difficulties not least in terms of where to look, what to measure, what values to assign to data and how to interpret results (Cobb 1998). It will also present the problem of comparability with other cases of need and the inevitable debate about resource allocation. These are issues that are generally left unspoken when attempting to support an holistic approach to care, but they are unavoidable issues when grounded in the practicalities of delivering a service to actual patients.

The perspective and experience of patients will be an essential part of research. There is an embarrassing absence of this perspective when considering spiritual care despite the inferences made from the most cursory of data collected from a patient upon admission: their 'religion'. Detailed case studies have the potential of providing a rich source for understanding this domain but they may be limited by the time required for their compilation; self-administered questionnaires, on the other hand, may result in a larger sample and a reduction in interviewer bias. Whatever the chosen method, the patients' perceptions will need to be elicited sensitively, particularly when the questioning depends upon the patients' understanding and acceptance of their prognosis. Questions posed to patients or their carers may induce anxiety or distress, cause unnecessary concern or disrupt the trust placed in carers. The art of designing questions which are psychometrically reliable and sensitive to patients will be one that is exercised considerably in pursuing research that involves the perspective of patients.

Finally, mention should be made of the need for effective dissemination of results to share significant findings, influence practice and nurture further research. This appears obvious until we examine the potential journals that may publish research in the spiritual domain, and then the possibility is diminished. It is difficult to know whether journals carry few research papers concerning spirituality because the research projects undertaken are few in number, poor in the quality of their design, or simply that spirituality is not a subject that enhances the reputation or sales of high-impact journals. Dissemination can be achieved by other means, but it is likely that similar issues will be a barrier to spirituality as an attractive research topic. It appears that spirituality has an uphill struggle as an area for research in palliative care but it is one which has the potential to achieve credibility and recognition.

Knowledge base

Spirituality is at first sight an ambiguous term open to a range of interpretation and meaning. The undetermined nature of spirituality is both appealing and daunting but it does not encourage a confident approach to the study and development of this domain. The spirituality of palliative care is less vague when considered from the historical perspective of the Christian faith which inspired the hospice movement. But the expansion and development of the movement and the shifting social context brought different philosophical perspectives to bear upon spirituality which became associated less with corporate religion and more with subjective experience. Perhaps the increasing spread of spirituality in palliative care reflects something of the widening notion and operation of what was once understood as a building, then a specialism and now an approach to care which reaches back to the point of diagnosis. Spirituality as a dimension of the philosophy of care has therefore had to adapt and be redefined to remain consistent with an increasingly inclusive and extensive understanding of palliative care.

The historical development of spirituality in palliative care has not generally been supported by developments in the knowledge base. On the surface there have been some indications of movement in this direction over such matters as definition and issues of policy and practice, but these have rarely addressed underlying concepts or epistemology. Mitigating reasons include the opposing assumptions that spirituality is a dangerously cavernous subject to try to understand or too irrational or ethereal to be subject to any study. It is also rare to find health professionals who have encountered spirituality as a subject in their training. All this leads away from the rigorous study of spirituality in the palliative care context unless an individual feels a strong personal motivation to pursue the subject.

Spirituality does not present a unitary field for study beyond a superficial or comparative level. It is not a single phenomenon but displays manifold forms that cut across a range of academic disciplines. In palliative care there are some boundaries that can be imposed and there are the evident foci of patients with life-threatening disease. The knowledge base is therefore eclectic but interrelated and draws upon well established traditions and schools. What palliative care has to bring to this knowledge base is experiential learning which can inform theory and provide the necessary dialectic for practice. A good example of this process is provided by the issue of euthanasia which draws together the patient, professional and public alongside such disciplines as moral philosophy, law and religion to contend with the question, 'What should be done?' Questions of what may be termed 'applied spirituality' locate abstract conceptual knowledge within experience and through their interaction promote mutual development.

The interdisciplinary and multidimensional approach advocated by palliative care would appear to provide a most conducive environment for the development of a knowledge base in spirituality. There is plentiful work to be undertaken among extant sources of knowledge and there is probably much to be gained from their creative interplay. The challenge is to provide effective opportunities to support such enterprise and to facilitate a wide critical enquiry. There is also the need for effective dialogue built upon mutual understanding and a respect for disciplines that may not usually be considered relevant or rigorous. The field is vast, some disciplines have staked various claims, but there is much open space. Suspicion and contempt will have to be overcome in some areas and there will certainly be a need for pioneers. The results can only be imagined at this stage, but the possibilities appear worthwhile to pursue.

Spiritual care

This final signpost is pointed towards the pragmatic issue of how spiritual care should be developed in practice. It is premised on the understanding that care is delivered by people trained to various levels to meet the needs of patients within a set of overarching goals and principles. A number of questions suggest themselves from this basic premise: what knowledge, attitudes and skills are required to practise spiritual care? How should these be taught and learnt? What counts as good spiritual care? How should spiritual care be incorporated into the models and practices of palliative care? As we find ourselves at the beginning of this exploration we can only begin to suggest what might be considered as possible answers to these major issues.

Spirituality is both a set of abstract concepts and concrete experience. In training health professionals to work in palliative care we will need to address the objective and subjective aspects of spirituality both of carer and of patient. Therefore it can be expected that cognitive and behavioural modes of learning will need to be complemented with experiential learning (Kolb 1993). First, however, there must be some agreement as to what is the nature of spiritual care and who should be involved in its provision – an area we have already noted as contentious. Research and the knowledge base will inform this process but there also needs to be local and national forums which provide the opportunity to move beyond propositional statements and engage with greater clarity in the practical issues that surround caring for people. This is not to suggest that spiritual care is waiting to be programmed into the delivery of palliative care as a uniform package across all settings. Nonetheless there are individual and organizational issues which need addressing to ensure a beneficial and reliable approach.

It is simplistic to suggest that spiritual care cannot be subject to standards and audit. Similarly it is naive to expect spiritual care to be reduced to a task-based operation. Between these two positions is to be found a proper concern for spiritual care that is sensitive to the limits of operational management whilst aware of the possibilities for promoting good practice. This requires a number of related areas to be addressed, including education, training, research and policy. The diversification of palliative care into a range of settings requires that the development of spiritual care is also attentive to its context and responsive to new initiatives. It seems reasonable to expect that this process has occurred locally to some extent; however, this remains only speculative without empirical evidence. In the absence of a lead body or without the concerted efforts of informed professionals, spiritual care will probably remain fragmentary and relatively coincidental to more strategically planned developments of palliative care services. This in itself may not be detrimental to spiritual care in particular settings, but it is unlikely to support the coordination of care across sites or the reduction of unacceptable variations in services.

In contrast to the broader developments in hospice and palliative care it would appear that the spiritual dimension has remained at an early developmental stage. There are many organizational and social reasons to explain this position, and some may contend that notions of progress or evolution are not appropriate to a matter that touches upon the eternal. Whilst there is some philosophical support for this insularity, the lived experience of patients and carers will ensure that spirituality is inextricably part of the whole and far from absent in the practical concerns of discerning and providing care. How palliative care services should respond to this aspect of living and dying is a question currently answered more by unexamined convention and assumption than by informed dialogue and enquiry. It remains to be seen how long this question goes unanswered by a specialism that has faced mortality in such a challenging and critical way.

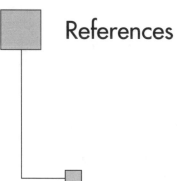

References

Ahmedzai, S., Hunt, J. and Keeley, V. (1998) *Palliative Care Core Standards*, 2nd edn. Sheffield: Trent Hospice Audit Group.

Ajemian, I. (1993) The interdisciplinary team, in D. Doyle, G.W.C. Hanks and N. MacDonald (eds) *Oxford Textbook of Palliative Medicine*. Oxford: Oxford University Press.

Autton, N. (1975) Pastoral care, in R.W. Raven (ed.) *The Dying Patient*. Kent: Pitman.

Badham, P. (1995) Death and immortality: towards a global synthesis, in D. Cohn-Sherbok and C. Lewis (eds) *Beyond Death*. Basingstoke: Macmillan.

Barnard, D. (1995) The promise of intimacy and the fear of our own undoing, *Journal of Palliative Care*, 11(4): 22–6.

Bauman, Z. (1998) Postmodern religion?, in P. Heelas (ed.) *Religion, Modernity and Postmodernity*. Oxford: Blackwell.

Beckford, J.A. and Gilliat, S. (1996) *The Church of England and Other Faiths in a Multi-faith Society*. Coventry: University of Warwick.

Beit-Hallahmi, B. and Argyle, M. (1997) *The Psychology of Religious Behaviour, Belief and Experience*. London: Routledge.

Berger, P.L. (1967) *The Sacred Canopy*. New York: Doubleday.

Berlins, I. (1996) *The Sense of Reality*. London: Chatto & Windus.

Blackmore, S. (1999) *The Meme Machine*. Oxford: Oxford University Press.

Bond, P. (1998) The primacy of theology and the question of perception, in P. Heelas (ed.) *Religion, Modernity and Postmodernity*. Oxford: Blackwell.

Bowker, J. (1983) *Worlds of Faith*. London: BBC.

Bowker, J. (1987) *Licensed Insanities*. London: Darton, Longman & Todd.

Bowker, J. (1991) *The Meanings of Death*. Cambridge: Cambridge University Press.

Bowker, J. (ed.) (1997) *The Oxford Dictionary of World Religions*. Oxford: Oxford University Press.

Bowling, A. (1997) *Research Methods in Health*. Buckingham: Open University Press.

Bown, J. and Williams, A. (1993) Spirituality and nursing: a review of the literature, *Journal of Advances in Health and Nursing Care*, 2(4): 41–66.

Bradshaw, A. (1996a) Lighting the lamp: the covenant as an encompassing framework for the spiritual dimension of nursing care, in E.S. Farmer (ed.) *Exploring the Spiritual Dimension in Caring*. Salisbury: Quay.

Bradshaw, A. (1996b) The spiritual dimension of hospice: secularization of an ideal, *Social Science and Medicine*, 43(3): 409–19.

Bradshaw, J. (1972) Taxonomy of social need, in G. McLachlan (ed.) *Problems and Progress in Medical Care*. London: Oxford University Press.

Bragan, K. (1996) *Self and Spirit in the Therapeutic Relationship*. London: Routledge.

Brierley, P. (ed.) (1997) *UK Christian Handbook: Religious Trends No.1 (1998/99 edn)*. London: Christian Research.

Brown, W.S., Murphy, N. and Newton Malony, H. (eds) (1998) *Whatever Happened to the Soul?* Minneapolis: Fortress Press.

Bruce, S. (1996) *Religion in the Modern World*. Oxford: Oxford University Press.

Calman, K. and Hine, D. (1995) *A Policy Framework for Commissioning Cancer Services*. London: Department of Health.

Campbell, A.V. (1984) *Moderated Love: A Theology of Professional Care*. London: SPCK.

Cant, S. and Sharmer, U. (1999) *A New Medical Pluralism?* London: UCL Press.

Cassel, E.J. (1982) The nature of suffering and the goals of medicine, *New England Journal of Medicine*, 306(11): 639–45.

Catterall, R.A., Cobb, M., Greet, B., Sankey, J. and Griffiths, G. (1998) The assessment and audit of spiritual care, *International Journal of Palliative Nursing*, 4(4): 162–8.

Cherry, C. (1995) Are near-death experiences really suggestive of life after death, in D. Cohn-Sherbok and C. Lewis (eds) *Beyond Death*. Basingstoke: Macmillan.

Cicirelli, V.G. (1998) Personal meanings of death in relation to fear of death, *Death Studies*, 22: 713–33.

Clark, C., Cross, J., Deane, D. and Lowry, L. (1991) Spirituality: integral to quality care, *Holistic Nursing Practice*, 5(3): 67–76.

Clark, D. (1998) Originating a movement: Cicely Saunders and the development of St Christopher's Hospice, 1957–1967, *Mortality*, 3(1): 43–63.

Clark, D. and Seymour, J. (1999) *Reflections on Palliative Care*. Buckingham: Open University Press.

Clarke, P. (1995) Beyond death: the case of new religions, in D. Cohn-Sherbok and C. Lewis (eds) *Beyond Death*. Basingstoke: Macmillan.

Cobb, M. (1998) Assessing spiritual needs: an examination of practice, in M. Cobb and V. Robshaw (eds) *The Spiritual Challenge of Health Care*. Edinburgh: Churchill Livingstone.

Corner, J. and Dunlop, R. (1997) New approaches to care, in D. Clark, J. Hockley and S. Ahmedzai (eds) *New Themes in Palliative Care*. Buckingham: Open University Press.

Cornette, K. (1997) For whenever I am weak, I am strong . . . , *International Journal of Palliative Nursing*, 3(1): 6–13.

Crabbe, M.J.C. (1999) *From Soul to Self*. London: Routledge.

Damasio, A. (1999) *The Feeling of What Happens: Body and Emotion in the Making of Consciousness*. London: William Heinemann.

Davie, G. (1994) *Religion in Britain since 1945*. Oxford: Blackwell.

Davies, D. (1996) The social facts of death, in G. Howarth and P.C. Jupp (eds) *Contemporary Issues in the Sociology of Death, Dying and Disposal*. Basingstoke: Macmillan.

Davies, D.J. (1997) *Death Ritual and Belief*. London: Cassell.

Davies, J.D. (1990) *Cremation Today and Tomorrow*. Nottingham: Grove.

Dawkins, R. (1995) *River out of Eden*. London: Weidenfeld & Nicolson.

Dein, S. and Stygall, J. (1997) Does being religious help or hinder coping with chronic illness? A critical literature review, *Palliative Medicine*, 11: 291–8.

Dudley, J., Smith, C. and Millison, M. (1995) Unfinished business: assessing the spiritual needs of hospice clients, *American Journal of Hospice and Palliative Care*, March/April.

Dunlop, R.J., Davies, R.J. and Hockley, J.M. (1989) Preferred versus actual place of death: a hospital palliative care support team experience, *Palliative Medicine*, 3: 197–201.

Dworkin, R. (1993) *Life's Dominion*. London: HarperCollins.

Elford, R.J. (1999) *The Pastoral Nature of Theology: An Upholding Presence*. London: Cassell.

Elsdon, R. (1995) Spiritual pain in dying people: the nurse's role, *Professional Nurse*, 10(10): 641–3.

Eraut, M. (1994) *Developing Professional Knowledge and Competence*. London: Falmer Press.

Flowers, B.S. (1998) Death, the bald scenario, in J. Malpas and R.C. Solomon (eds) *Death and Philosophy*. London: Routledge.

Fulton, R. (1986) Commentary, in F.S. Wald (ed.) *In Quest of the Spiritual Component of Care for the Terminally Ill*. New Haven, CT: Yale University School of Nursing.

Gadamer, H-G. (1996) *The Enigma of Health*. Cambridge: Polity Press.

Gallop, D. (ed. and trans.) (1993) *Phaedo*. Oxford: Oxford University Press.

George, R. and Sykes, J. (1997) Beyond cancer?, in D. Clark, J. Hockley and S. Ahmedzai (eds) *New Themes in Palliative Care*. Buckingham: Open University Press.

Gerkin, C.V. (1997) *An Introduction to Pastoral Care*. Nashville, TN: Abingdon.

Gibbs, L.M.E., Addington-Hall, J. and Gibbs, J.S.R. (1998) Dying from heart failure: lessons from palliative care, *British Medical Journal*, 317: 961–2.

Giddens, A. (1990) *The Consequences of Modernity*. Stanford, CA: Stanford University Press.

Gillon, R. (1985) *Philosophical Medical Ethics*. London: Wiley/British Medical Journal.

Glickman, M. (1996) *Palliative Care in the Hospital Setting*, occasional paper no. 10. London: National Council for Hospice and Specialist Palliative Care Services.

Glickman, M. (1997) *Making Palliative Care Better*, occasional paper no. 12. London: National Council for Hospice and Specialist Palliative Care Services.

Golsworthy, R. and Coyle, A. (1999) Spiritual beliefs and the search for meaning among older adults following partner loss, *Mortality*, 4(1): 21–40.

Goodliff, P. (1998) *Care in a Confused Climate: Pastoral Care and Postmodern Culture*. London: Darton, Longman & Todd.

Grey, A. (1994) The spiritual component of palliative care, *Palliative Medicine*, 8: 215–21.

Griffin, J. (1986) *Well-being*. Oxford: Oxford University Press.

Gunaratnam, Y. (1997) Culture is not enough, in D. Field, J. Hockey and N. Small (eds) *Death, Gender and Ethnicity*. London: Routledge.

Hallam, E., Hockey, J. and Howarth, G. (1999) *Beyond the Body: Death and Social Identity*. London: Routledge.

Hammarskjöld, D. (1964) *Markings*. London: Faber & Faber.

Hare, D. (1995) *Skylight*. London: Faber & Faber.

Hay, D. (1982) *Exploring Inner Space*. London: Penguin.

Heaven, C.M. and Maguire, P. (1997) Disclosure of concerns by hospice patients and their identification by nurses, *Palliative Medicine*, 11: 283–90.

Heelas, P. (1996) *The New Age Movement*. Oxford: Blackwell.

Heyes-Moore, L.H. (1996) On spiritual pain in the dying, *Mortality* 1(3): 297–315.

Hick, J. (1999) *The Fifth Dimension: An Exploration of the Spiritual Realm*. Oxford: Oneworld.

Hill, D. and Penso, D. (1997) *Opening Doors*, occasional paper no. 7. London: National Council for Hospice and Specialist Palliative Care Services.

Hill, S. (1998) *The Service of Clouds*. London: Chatto & Windus.

Holland, J.C., Paasik, S., Kash, K.A. *et al.* (1999) The role of religious and spiritual beliefs in coping with malignant melanoma, *Psycho-Oncology*, 8: 14–26.

Illich, I. (1976) *Limits to Medicine*. London: Penguin.

Jacobs, M. (1993) *Living Illusions*. London: SPCK.

Jacobs, M. (1998) Faith as the 'space between', in M. Cobb and V. Robshaw (eds) *The Spiritual Challenge of Health Care*. Edinburgh: Churchill Livingstone.

Johnson, G. (1995) *Fire in the Mind*. London: Viking.

Jung, C. (1933) *Modern Man in Search of a Soul*. London: Routledge.

Keizer, B. (1997) *Dancing with Mister D*. London: Black Swan.

Kerr, F. (1997) *Immortal Longings*. London: SPCK.

King, M., Speck, P. and Thomas, A. (1994) Spiritual and religious beliefs in acute illness, *Social Science and Medicine*, 38: 4.

King, M., Speck, P. and Thomas, A. (1999) The effect of spiritual beliefs on outcome from illness, *Social Science and Medicine* 48: 1291–9.

Klemke, E.D. (2000) *The Meaning of Life*, 2nd edn. New York: Oxford University Press.

Koehn, D. (1994) *The Ground of Professional Ethics*. London: Routledge.

Koenig, H.G., Cohen, H.J., Blazer, H.J. *et al.* (1992) Religious coping and depression among elderly, hospitalized medically ill men, *American Journal of Psychiatry*, 149(12): 1693–700.

Kogan, M. and Redfern, S. (1995) *Making Use of Clinical Audit*. Buckingham: Open University Press.

Kolb, D.A. (1993) The process of experiential learning, in M. Thorpe, R. Edwards and A. Hanson (eds) *Culture and Processes of Adult Learning*. London: Routledge.

Lake, F. (1986) *Clinical Theology*. London: Darton, Longman & Todd.

LeDoux, J. (1998) *The Emotional Brain*. London: Weidenfeld & Nicolson.

Llewellyn, N. (1991) *The Art of Death*. London: Reaktion/Victoria and Albert Museum.

Lucas, J.R. (1993) *Responsibility*. Oxford: Oxford University Press.
Lyall, D. (1995) *Counselling in the Pastoral and Spiritual Context*. Buckingham: Open University Press.
Lyall, D. (1998) Pastoral integrity, ethical reflection and hospital politics, *Journal of Health Care Chaplaincy*, October: 17–26.
Lynch, T. (1998) *The Undertaking*. London: Vintage.
Lyon, D. (1996) Religion and the postmodern: old problems, new prospects, in K. Flanagan and P. Jupp (eds) *Postmodernity, Sociology and Religion*. Basingstoke: Macmillan.
Markham, I. (1998) Spirituality and the world faiths, in M. Cobb and V. Robshaw (eds) *The Spiritual Challenge of Health Care*. Edinburgh: Churchill Livingstone.
Marris, P. (1986) *Loss and Change*. London: Routledge.
Martin, P. (1997) *The Sickening Mind*. London: HarperCollins.
Maxwell, R.J. (1984) Quality assessment in health, *British Medical Journal*, 288: 1470–1.
McGrath, P. (1998) Buddhist spirituality – a compassionate perspective on hospice care, *Mortality*, 3(3): 251–63.
Mellor, P. (1993) Death in high modernity: the contemporary presence and absence of death, in D. Clark (ed.) *The Sociology of Death*. Oxford: Blackwell.
Mills, S. and Peacock, W. (1997) *Professional Organisation of Complementary and Alternative Medicine in the United Kingdom 1997*. Exeter: University of Exeter.
Mitterrand, F. (1997) Foreword, in M. De Hennezel, *Intimate Death*. London: Warner Books.
Morea, P. (1997) *In Search of Personality*. London: SCM.
Muir, E. (1997) *Ritual in Early Modern Europe*. Cambridge: Cambridge University Press.
NCHSPCS (1995) *Specialist Palliative Care: A Statement of Definitions*, occasional paper no. 8. London: National Council for Hospice and Specialist Palliative Care Services.
NCHSPCS (1996) *Education in Palliative Care*, occasional paper no. 9. London: National Council for Hospice and Specialist Palliative Care Services.
Neimeyer, R.A. (1997) Death anxiety research: the state of the art, *Omega*, 36(2): 97–120.
Nelson, J. (1992) *The Intimate Connection*. London: SPCK.
Neuberger, J. (1999) *Dying Well: A Guide to Enabling a Good Death*. Hale: Hochland & Hochland.
Nicholson, K. (1997) *Body and Soul: The Transcendence of Materialism*. Colorado: Westview Press.
Nuland, S.B. (1994) *How We Die*. London: Chatto & Windus.
Okri, B. (1997) *A Way of Being Free*. London: Phoenix House.
Oldnall, A. (1996) A critical analysis of nursing: meeting the spiritual needs of patients, *Journal of Advance Nursing*, 23: 138–44.
Paterson, D. (1999) *The Eyes*. London: Faber & Faber.
Pattison, S. (1996) Should pastoral care have aims and objectives?, *Contact*, 20: 26–34.
Pattison, S. (1997) *The Faith of the Managers*. London: Cassell.
Pellegrino, E.D. and Thomasma, D.C. (1988) *For the Patient's Good*. New York: Oxford University Press.

Polkinghorne, J. (1996) *Beyond Science*. Cambridge: Cambridge University Press.

Porter, R. (1997) *The Greatest Benefit to Mankind*. London: HarperCollins.

Potter, D. (1994) *Seeing the Blossom*. London: Faber & Faber.

Randall, F. and Downie, R.S. (1996) *Palliative Care Ethics*. Oxford: Oxford University Press.

Rappaport, R.A. (1999) *Ritual and Religion in the Making of Humanity*. Cambridge: Cambridge University Press.

Reed, P.G. (1992) An emerging paradigm for the investigation of spirituality in nursing, *Research in Nursing and Health*, 15: 349–57.

Richman, C. (1994) I will keep the light, in B. Kirkpatrick (ed.) *Cry Love, Cry Hope*. London: Darton, Longman & Todd.

Roper, N., Logan, W. and Tierney Reader, A.J. (1996) *The Elements of Nursing*. Edinburgh: Churchill Livingstone.

Rose, G. (1995) *Love's Work*. London: Chatto & Windus.

Rose, G. (1996) *Mourning Becomes the Law*. Cambridge: Cambridge University Press.

Ross, L.A. (1994) Spiritual aspects of nursing, *Journal of Advance Nursing*, 19: 439–47.

Sacks, O. (1982) *Awakenings*. London: Picador.

Sartre, J-P. ([1946] 1997) *Existentialism and Humanism*. London: Methuen.

Saunders, C. (1988) Spiritual pain, *Hospital Chaplain*, March.

Schön, D.A. (1987) *Educating the Reflective Practitioner*. San Francisco: Jossey-Bass.

Scott Holland, H. (1919) *Facts of Faith*. London: Longman.

Scruton, R. (1996) *An Intelligent Person's Guide to Philosophy*. London: Duckworth.

Scruton, R. (1998) *An Intelligent Person's Guide to Modern Culture*. London: Duckworth.

Seale, C. (1998) *Constructing Death*. Cambridge: Cambridge University Press.

Smaje, C. and Field, D. (1997) Absent minorities? Ethnicity and the use of palliative care services, in D. Field, J. Hockey, and N. Small (eds) *Death, Gender and Ethnicity*. London: Routledge.

Small, N. (1998) Spirituality and hospice care, in M. Cobb and V. Robshaw (eds) *The Spiritual Challenge of Health Care*. Edinburgh: Churchill Livingstone.

Smart, N. (1989) *The World's Religions*. Cambridge: Cambridge University Press.

Smart, N. (1996) *Dimensions of the Sacred*. London: HarperCollins.

Soll, I. (1998) On the purported insignificance of death, in J. Malpas and R.C. Solomon (eds) *Death and Philosophy*. London: Routledge.

Solomon, R.C. (1998) Death fetishism, morbid solipsism, in J. Malpas and R.C. Solomon (eds) *Death and Philosophy*. London: Routledge.

Sontag, S. (1991) *Illness as Metaphor/Aids and its Metaphors*. London: Penguin.

Speck, P. (1998) Spiritual issues in palliative care, in D. Doyle, G.W.C. Hanks and N. MacDonald (eds) *Oxford Textbook of Palliative Medicine*. Oxford: Oxford University Press.

Stoddard, S. (1979) *The Hospice Movement: A Better Way of Caring for the Dying*. London: Jonathan Cape.

Stoter, D. (1995) *Spiritual Aspects of Health Care*. London: Mosby.

Swinburne, R. (1997) *The Evolution of the Soul*. Oxford: Oxford University Press.

Taylor, E.J., Amenta, M. and Highfield, M. (1995) Spiritual care practices of oncology nurses, *Oncology Nursing Forum*, 22(1): 31–9.

Thomas, R.S. (1995) *Collected Poems 1945–1990*. London: J.M. Dent.

Thrower, J. (1999) *Religion: The Classical Theories*. Edinburgh: Edinburgh University Press.

Tilby, A. (1992) *Science and the Soul*. London: SPCK.

Tillich, P. (1952) *The Courage to Be*. New Haven, CT: Yale University Press.

Tomer, A. and Eliason, G. (1996) Toward a comprehensive model of death anxiety, *Death Studies*, 20: 343–65.

Trías, E. (1998) Thinking religion: the symbol and the sacred, in J. Derrida and G. Vattimo (eds) *Religion*. Stanford, CA: Stanford University Press.

Twycross, R.G. and Lack, S.A. (1990) *Therapeutics in Terminal Cancer*. Edinburgh: Churchill Livingstone.

Wald, F.S. (ed.) (1986) *In Quest of the Spiritual Component of Care for the Terminally Ill*. New Haven, CT: Yale University School of Nursing.

Walter, T. (1997) The ideology and organization of spiritual care: three approaches, *Palliative Medicine*, 11: 21–30.

Walter, T. (1999) *On Bereavement: The Culture of Grief*. Buckingham: Open University Press.

Ward, K. (1992) *Defending the Soul*. Oxford: Oneworld.

Weller, P. (1997) *Religions in the UK*. Derby: University of Derby.

Wertheim, M. (1999) *The Pearly Gates of Cyberspace*. London: Virago.

Wilcock, P. (1996) *Spiritual Care of Dying and Bereaved People*. London: SPCK.

Wilde, O. (1986) *De Profundis and Other Writings*. London: Penguin.

Wilson, A.N. (1995) Life after death, in D. Cohn-Sherbok and C. Lewis (eds) *Beyond Death*. Basingstoke: Macmillan.

Worden, J.W. (1991) *Grief Counselling and Grief Therapy*. London: Routledge.

Worden, J.W. (1996) *Children and Grief*. New York: Guilford.

Working Party on the Impact of Hospice Experience on the Church's Ministry of Healing (1991) *Mud and Stars*. Oxford: Sobell.

Wright, F. (1996) *Pastoral Care Revisited*. London: SCM.

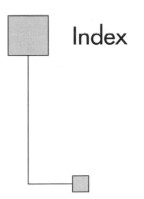

Index

AN INTIMATE LONELINESS
SUPPORTING BEREAVED PARENTS AND SIBLINGS

Gordon Riches and Pam Dawson

- What impact does a child's death have on family relationships?
- How might differences in the way mothers and fathers deal with bereavement contribute to increased marital tension?
- Why are bereaved siblings so deeply affected by the way their parents grieve?

An Intimate Loneliness explores how family members attempt to come to terms with the death of an offspring or brother or sister. Drawing on relevant research and the authors' own experience of working with bereaved parents and siblings, this book examines the importance of social relationships in helping them adjust to their bereavement. The chances of making sense of this most distressing loss are influenced by the resilience of the family's surviving relationships, by the availability of wider support networks and by the cultural resources that inform each's perception of death. This book considers the impact of bereavement on self and family identity. In particular, it examines the role of shared remembering in transforming survivor's relationships with the deceased, and in helping rebuild their own identity with a significantly changed family structure. Problems considered include: the failure of intimate relationships, cultural and gender expectations, the 'invisibility' of fathers' and siblings' grief, sudden and 'difficult' deaths, lack of information, and the sense of isolation felt by some family members.

This book will be of value to students on courses in counselling, health care, psychology, social policy, pastoral care and education. It will appeal to sociology students with an interest in death, dying and mortality. It is also aimed at professionally qualified counselling, health and social service workers, informed voluntary group members, the clergy, teachers and others involved with pastoral care.

Contents
Introduction – Order out of chaos: personal, social and cultural resources for making sense of loss – A bleak and lonely landscape: problems of adjustment for bereaved parents – What about me? Problems of adjustment for bereaved siblings – Connections and disconnections: ways family members deal with lost relationships – Difficult deaths and problems of adjustment – Things that help: supporting bereaved parents and brothers and sisters – Conclusion: professional support in a post-modern world – Appendix: shoe-strings and bricolage: some notes on the background research project

240pp   0 335 19972 0 (Paperback)   0 335 19973 9 (Hardback)

ON BEREAVEMENT
THE CULTURE OF GRIEF

Tony Walter

Insightful and refreshing.
> Professor Dennis Klass, Webster University, St Louis, USA

A tour de force.
> Dr Colin Murray Parkes, OBE, MD, FRCPsych,
> President of CRUSE

Some societies and some individuals find a place for their dead, others leave them behind. In recent years, researchers, professionals and bereaved people themselves have struggled with this. Should the bond with the dead be continued or broken? What is clear is that the grieving individual is not left in a social vacuum but has to struggle with expectations from self, family, friends, professionals and academic theorists.

This ground-breaking book looks at the social position of the bereaved. They find themselves caught between the living and the dead, sometimes searching for guidelines in a de-ritualized society that has few to offer, sometimes finding their grief inappropriately pathologized and policed. At its best, bereavement care offers reassurance, validation and freedom to talk where the client has previously encountered judgmentalism.

In this unique book, Tony Walter applies sociological insights to one of the most personal of human situations. *On Bereavement* is aimed at students on medical, nursing, counselling and social work courses that include bereavement as a topic. It will also appeal to sociology students with an interest in death, dying and mortality.

Contents
Introduction – Part I: Living with the dead – Other places, other times – War, peace and the dead: twentieth-century popular culture – Private bonds – Public bonds: the dead in everyday conversation – The last chapter – Theories – Part II: Policing grief – Guidelines for grief: historical background – Popular guidelines: the English case – Expert guidelines: clinical lore – Vive la différence? The politics of gender – Bereavement care – Conclusion: integration, regulation and postmodernism – References – Index.

256pp   0 335 20080 X (Paperback)   0 335 20081 8 (Hardback)

REFLECTIONS ON PALLIATIVE CARE

David Clark and Jane Seymour

Palliative care seems set to continue its rapid development into the early years of the twenty-first century. From its origins in the modern hospice movement, the new multidisciplinary specialty of palliative care has expanded into a variety of settings. Palliative care services are now being provided in the home, in hospital and in nursing homes. There are moves to extend palliative care beyond its traditional constituency of people with cancer. Efforts are being made to provide a wide range of palliative therapies to patients at an early stage of their disease progression. The evidence-base of palliative care is growing, with more research, evaluation and audit, along with specialist programmes of education. Palliative care appears to be coming of age.

On the other hand numbers of challenges still exist. Much service development has been unplanned and unregulated. Palliative care providers must continue to adapt to changing patterns of commissioning and funding services. The voluntary hospice movement may feel its values threatened by a new professionalism and policies which require its greater integration within mainstream services. There are concerns about the re-medicalization of palliative care, about how an evidence-based approach to practice can be developed, and about the extent to which its methods are transferring across diseases and settings.

Beyond these preoccupations lie wider societal issues about the organization of death and dying in late modern culture. To what extent have notions of death as a contemporary taboo been superseded? How can we characterize the nature of suffering? What factors are involved in the debate surrounding end of life care ethics and euthanasia?

David Clark and Jane Seymour, drawing on a wide range of sources, as well as their own empirical studies, offer a set of reflections on the development of palliative care and its place within a wider social context. Their book will be essential reading to any practitioner, policy maker, teacher or student involved in palliative care or concerned about death, dying and life-limiting illness.

Contents
Introduction – Part 1: Death in society – The social meaning of death and suffering – Ageing, dying and grieving – The ethics of dying – Part II: The philosophy and practice of palliative care – History and development – Definitions, components, meanings – Routinization and medicalization – Part III: Policy issues – Policy development and palliative care – The delivery of palliative care services – Part IV: Conclusion – The future for palliative care – References – Index.

224pp   0 335 19454 0 (Paperback)   0 335 19455 9 (Hardback)

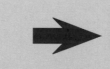